Janice Zarro Brodman, PhD

Sex RULES!

Astonishing
SEXUAL PRACTICES AND GENDER ROLES
AROUND THE WORLD

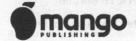

mango
PUBLISHING

Published by Mango Publishing Group, a division of Mango Media Inc.

Cover Design: Michele Shortley

Layout & Design: Morgane Leoni

For permission requests, please contact the publisher at:

Mango Publishing Group

2850 Douglas Road, 3rd Floor

Coral Gables, FL 33134 USA

info@mango.bz

For special orders, quantity sales, course adoptions and corporate sales, please email the publisher at sales@mango.bz. For trade and wholesale sales, please contact Ingram Publisher Services at customer.service@ingramcontent.com or +1.800.509.4887.

Sex Rules!

Library of Congress Cataloging-in-Publication number: 2017909204

ISBN: (paperback) 978-1-63353-593-0 , (ebook) 978-1-63353-594-7

BISAC category code PER004010 PERFORMING ARTS / Film & Video / Direction & Production

Printed in the United States of America

Praise for Sex Rules!

"Toss your preconceptions overboard and jump on a wild tour of 'No-way!' sexual customs, LOL gender switcheroos, and plenty of eye-popping moments. This is the world's weirdest and funniest reality show. But it's more. It's fascinating and smart, and all true. It will give you a new way of looking at the world. And when you feel your most bizarre, it offers a comforting lesson: You're not alone! There's a place in this world for everyone."

> –Richard Bangs, often called "the Father of Modern Adventure Travel," led "firsts" in travel worldwide, writes for HuffingtonPost.com, produces and hosts the National Public TV series *Richard Bangs' Adventures with Purpose*. He blogs on *Quests: Keep the Quest Alive* (http://www.richardbangs.com)

"It's a scientific fact! Women have better orgasms with funny partners. Read this hilarious book and you'll have more and better sex, happier relationships and a healthier libido! Quote it to friends and you'll never be lonely. And if your lover/boss/parent/spouse catches you doubled over, gasping with laughter, just look superior and say you've taken up anthropology."

> –Joanne Sandler, former Deputy Executive Director of the UN Development Fund for Women (UNIFEM), is

a senior associate of Gender@Work, an international collaborative that strengthens organizations to build cultures of equality and social justice. She co-produces the popular podcast *Two Old Bitches*. (http://www.twooldbitches.com/)

"From its first pages, *Sex Rules! Astonishing Sexual Practices and Gender Roles Around the World* opens a door onto a page-turning world rich with variety, humor and unexpected twists of sexual practices around the world. It's fresh, intriguing and of course titillating. But it's also thought-provoking and timely. We in the Western world have locked sex into norms only now being challenged on so many levels. This book's look at diverse world cultures and their 'acceptable' sexual practice is fascinating, often funny in the telling, and deeply surprising. I highly recommend *Sex Rules!* to anyone who has a hunger to delve into rarely seen corners of the world, enjoy a good laugh, and learn from a trained scholar as she takes you on this journey that reveals 'Sex Rules' in all their staggering variety."

—Ed Robbins is an award-winning Director-Writer-Producer and Digital Journalist. His programs have aired on PBS, Discovery Channel, TLC, Nat Geo Channel, ABC, NBC, BBC2 and Channel 4; his stories have been published in the *NY Times, Time Magazine,* and the International Reporting Project. He's an Adjunct Professor at Columbia University.

"The world needs more laughs, more fun, wider caring and understanding. Enter, this book. Yes, it's very funny, but it's so much more. Stunning facts about intriguing cultures you didn't even know exist – and may not much longer. 'Weird' cultures that give insights into our own. The author clearly likes and respects these folks, who seem strange from our POV but have their own logic. She tackles sexism, dogmatism, and intolerance with that powerful force: marvelous humor."

–Isa Maria Infante, Ph.D., J.D., Green Party candidate for Governor of Tennessee, former dean at SUNY, leader of Sugar Tree Bluegrass, an all-women's bluegrass band, playwright and performer of her international one-woman show, *Las Cucarachas*.

Acknowledgements

My deepest thanks to my family, who inspire and delight me, to Isa, who helped create the book's initial concept, and most of all to Stuart, whose support and curiosity have made life a pleasure and this book possible.

Contents

Marriage and Other Mysteries   111

Foxy Lad(y) or Dress for Success   153

Introduction

"Normal sex." Clear what it is, right?

Think again.

India, Ghana, Tunisia, Mali...dozens of countries, hundreds of cultures, and everywhere I go, people are curious.

"What do they wear in Ladakh?" they ask.

"What's the food like in Ghana?"

"What do they do for fun in Suriname?"

Just one thing they never ask—because they figure sex is the same everywhere.

I know better...

I learned about weird sex at Harvard University. Not from a dirty old professor or horny undergrad, but from Tozzer, the Harvard Anthropology Library. I sat, drowsy and bored in the dim, silent Tozzer Reading Room. What demon convinced me to take anthropology? *Pentadactylism... avunculocal...durophagy...* Who makes up this crap?

Suddenly, my eyes shot open.

Hey, I'm from New Jersey. I *know* about weird sex. But...

Husbands who fret if their wives don't have enough lovers...? Teenagers *required* to take as many sex partners as possible...? Societies where all agree that *every* man should have a male lover...?

It was a goldmine of screwball sex, flipped-out mating. All hidden under stodgy anthropology garble.

It became a hobby. Fascinating, hilarious, astounding and—let's face it—*weird* sex and gender rules and roles around the world. I could send people into hysterics, shock the most jaded, amaze the sophisticates.

"You're kidding!" friends would scream. "I don't believe it! They *couldn't*!"

But they could. They did. They **do.**

Sure, sometimes it seemed *too much*. But I don't relish eating insects either, though millions of people love them. For me, the lesson was: no one way works for everyone— even for sex. If it doesn't harm or endanger anyone, no need to *adopt* the differences, but do *respect* them. Just be smart. It really does take a village to raise a child.

So if your lover complains your sex-play should be in Ripley's *Believe It Or Not*...

Your mom reveals her stash of kinky sex toys...

Dad's been modeling your favorite dress...

Rejoice!

There are places in this world where your most depraved fantasies would be considered tame. Where Grandma's idea of normal would drive the neighbors wild. Where your most wanton desires are simply part of daily life.

When it comes to sex, our human family is endlessly inventive. So celebrate! Make *your own* best rules. How about this one: Sex is fun!

Sex,
LIES AND
VIRGINS' TASTES
OR HOW TO PICK
A LOVER

I headed to India as a student in the '70s. The sexual revolution had declared victory back home in Boston. Sleeping with an attractive stranger was *de rigueur*. Living with your lover was expected. Sex before marriage the rule. They were the innocent days before HIV/AIDS.

Never before more than two hundred miles from home, I flew from Boston to Athens, crossed Greece, Turkey, Iran, Afghanistan, Pakistan, and India by motor boat, ferry, train, bus, and hippie van. A free spirit!

My first bias, and the most wrong-headed, was that people everywhere are pretty much the same. I wasn't a total fool. I knew some things would be different, like what you ate and how you dressed. I knew dating was forbidden in most countries. Parents arranged marriages, rarely with a woman's input or assent.

I knew I'd have to adjust. Just not how much.

Early on, near the Red Sea, I took refuge from the sun beneath the canopy of a Moroccan family's tent. I spoke no Arabic and they no English, so I held sketchy conversations with the mother in my shaky French. I must have made a good impression, because she soon asked how they could contact my parents. She announced—with an indulgent smile—that she and her husband decided to marry her son to me. Sitting nearby, he flushed, astonished. Obviously, no one had consulted him. The bride-price, she declared confidently: eighteen camels and six goats. Surely my parents couldn't refuse.

I stuttered in fractured French: It was very generous of her, and of course I was delighted. But I—not my parents—would decide whom I'd marry. Although I liked her very much and thought her son quite handsome (I could say nothing of his intelligence and wit, as he'd been mute the entire afternoon), I was not prepared to marry him or anyone else.

She was patently skeptical.

The next day, I was pleased with my skillful handling of another culture. It didn't take long to realize I didn't have a clue. The extremes I was about to experience—in every direction—would enrage, awe, humble, and sometimes terrify me.

Weeks later, in Afghanistan, I entered another world. Even pre-Taliban, the women were specters eclipsed in full-length black cloth, their eyes trapped behind dark grilles. Despite the glaring heat, I had dressed carefully in a dark, shapeless, long-sleeved shirt, a loose, black, ankle-length skirt, and a scarf covering my hair. I was as sexy as a sack of rice.

Much good it did. When the public bus from Kandahar to Kabul stopped so we passengers could relieve ourselves, I followed the local custom and found a boulder that I could squat behind in "private."

The man who jumped me was sure that I wouldn't scream, and, even if I did, no one would respond. When I jabbed an elbow into his chest he dropped his hold, more out of astonishment than pain, as if, about to bite into a potato, it had shoved him away. I ran.

It was my first gut-level experience of women's subjugation to men, but not my last. That many men expect, and get, utter compliance, was no great shock—except to my self-assurance.

Equally astonishing, and far happier, were the opposite experiences. They transformed everything I "knew" about women and men. Women ruling the seduction game, aggressively wooing coquettish men, setting (and resetting) the terms of marriage—were a revelation. "Normal" mating took on a whole new meaning as I came to know my neighbors around the globe.

Is that a vibrator in your pocket, or are you glad to see me?

Who's more obsessed with sex, men or women? Now there's a no-brainer, declare the Biwat of Papua New Guinea: *Women!*

Women, they explain, are ruled by uncontrollable lust. No normal woman can smother her incessant, raging desire for sex...much less wait for marriage.

Papua New Guinea is crazy diverse, with over 850 totally different societies in a country the size of California. The Biwat live deep in PNG's rainforest and swamps, in tiny villages along the fertile banks of the Yuat River. The main crop is betel, a lovely little drug plant that gives a nice buzz, boosts energy, and enjoys a thriving market in towns. The Biwat themselves don't use betel much. They have better things to do.

Though the men claim to want only virgins, young Biwat women polish their skin with oil, dress in their sexiest grass skirts, and are constantly cruising for new lovers— even after they are engaged to be married. See someone cute in his flying foxskin loincloth nicely decorated with shells? Getting to know him well enough for a roll in the woods takes about three seconds. As long as she's even the slightest bit discreet, everyone happily ignores her little lapses.

Want to know which guy got lucky? Easy. Fresh bite wounds around the neck, ripped clothes, face and arms scratched and bleeding.

The Biwat easily explain a woman's wild sexual antics: "Has she not a vulva?"

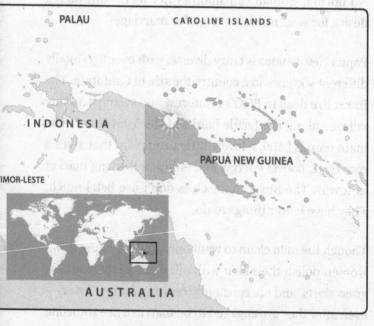

BIWAT OF PAPUA NEW GUINEA

Make love, not war

In Mangaian legend, the first human rose from a hole in the center of this lovely green Polynesian Island. Mangaia (*A'ua'u Enua*), which means "peace," is lush with tropical fruit, has plentiful, clean water, and no poisonous snakes or dangerous insects.

Mangaians learn early that life is sweet. Best of all, as they grow older, kids realize they have the world's greatest built-in entertainment: their genitals. No Mangaian would be so stupid as to call them "private" parts. All good parents encourage their growing kids to take advantage of the gifts nature gave them and masturbate.

Societies create lots of words for things they think important. Mangaians enjoy a wide vocabulary for the aesthetics of the clitoris: how large, pointed, pendulous, protruding, sharp, straight, and so on. The typical Mangaian male knows more about female genitals than most Western doctors.

Mangaians believe anything worth doing is worth learning to do well. As a boy enters mid-teens, he gets a tutor—an older, experienced woman, who teaches him a wide variety of positions, coaches him on how to use oral sex for best effect, and trains him in the skills that will arouse his partner and drown her in pleasure. His goal: to bring his partner to orgasm as many times as possible.

Mid-teen girls also receive a proper education. Their training focuses on how to have multiple intense orgasms. Needless to say, *all* Mangaian women are orgasmic.

Women score their lovers and broadcast which guy has good technique. One test is whether he can bring her to orgasm without touching anything except her vagina. A man must give his partner at least three orgasms before his own, or he's a loser. Then it's: Shape up, sugar, or it's back to masturbation.

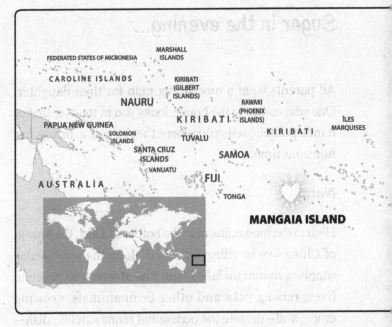

MANGAIA ISLAND

Sugar in the evening...

All parents want a nice young man for their daughter. One who comes to the house, looks you in the eye, shakes hands politely, tells you where they're going, brings her home on time.

Not...

High in the mountains near the border of Tibet, the Mosuo of China live in villages nestled along the spectacular sapphire mountain lake Lugu. The Mosuo lead peaceful lives, raising yaks and other farm animals, growing crops, and—despite the occasional home satellite dish—following tradition.

They call the late teen years the "honey time." At sixteen, a girl gets complete freedom to "make friends" with boys; that is, invite a chosen boy to spend the night in her bedroom in a special *Azhu* house. A girl is free to "make friends" with as many boys as she likes, and she alone decides what boy she'll befriend.

When the girl decides the romance is over, she simply shuts the door of her *Azhu* house to him.

There's just one fixed rule: the boy must show unfailing respect for her mother. He does it by sneaking into the girl's bedroom after dark, when Mom's asleep, and slipping out again before dawn, so no one will see him.

A boy who dares to show up in daylight to meet a girl's parents proves he's a disrespectful scoundrel with no respect for propriety...and Mom will toss him out on his sorry ass.

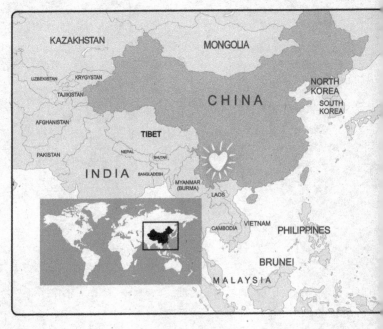

MOSUO OF CHINA

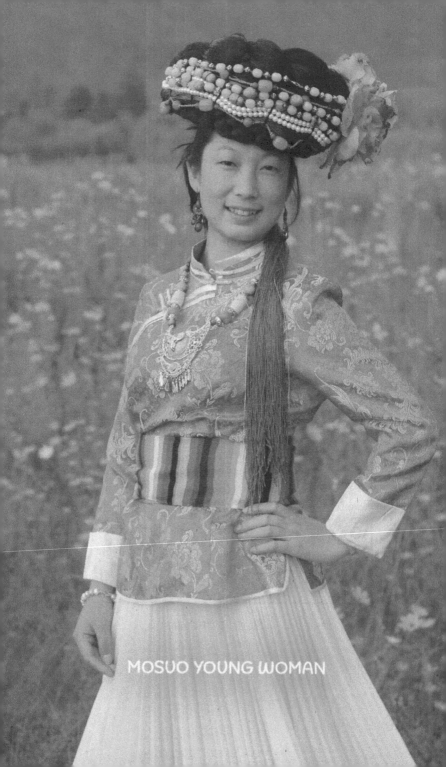

MOSUO YOUNG WOMAN

WEIRD SEX LAWS

Think it's odd that governments try to regulate something as ubiquitous, personal, and diverse as sex? Probably, but that's never stopped them. Take the USA. It has more laws regulating sex than all of Europe. Some laws make sense, of course. They protect the innocent. Others are just... weird.

If necrophilia is your thing, head to one of the states where it's legal: Louisiana, North Carolina, Oklahoma, Kansas, Missouri, and Wisconsin.

But be careful about getting it on with the living. In Connecticut, one old law forbade any "private sexual behavior between consenting adults" – that apparently included married couples.

Not to be outdone, Virginia outlaws exposing your genitals where anyone else is present – that includes in your bedroom with your lover. They can also lock you up for having sex with another consenting adult – or masturbating in someone else's presence. For those evil crimes, you can get twelve months in the hoosegow and a $2,500 fine.

Let's not forget an old law in Washington State that forbids intercourse with a virgin. No one gets away with flouting this law, including newlyweds. The penalties include prison and a fine.

Clawson, Michigan made it illegal for a farmer to sleep with his pigs, cows, horses, goats, and chickens. Now what will Clawson guys do on those long winter nights?

In the liberated state of Florida, it's illegal for a man to kiss his wife's breasts.

Colorado made it illegal to kiss a sleeping woman.

Florida staunchly protects its porcupines' virtue. Any human caught having sexual relations with a porcupine will face the full fury of the law, not to mention some major private parts pain.

In Illinois, they prohibit you from nuzzling or kissing a reptile.

Last but certainly not least, in liberated Massachusetts, the town of Salem has taken a firm stand. They made it illegal for married couples to sleep nude together in a rented room.

Don't yap about your yoni

On the isle of Yap, in Micronesia, surrounded by vast coral reefs and crystal-clear waters, people pursue age-old pastimes. Fishing, sailing, and weaving are still the center of daily life. Yap women preserve another tradition. They carefully guard the source of all their potency: their genitals. That way, they always have plenty of "power" to catch and hold any men they want.

No Yap woman would ever let *any* other female—young or old—get a peek at the source of her competitive edge, her *yoni*. They think Western women who go to female doctors are nuts. After all, a female doc is just as dangerous as any other woman. Who knows what the sneaky doc would snatch under cover of the exam room?

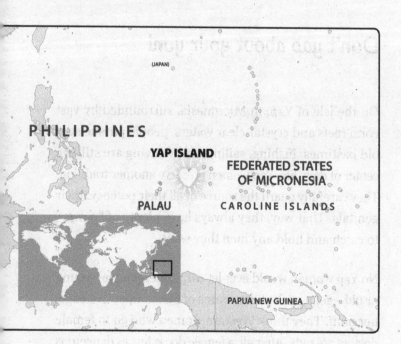

YAP ISLAND

Real dirty dancing...

Love to dance but got no partner? Come join the *Wayuu!* They are a happy lot. And for good reason. They wander freely through the jungles, deserts, and beautiful Caribbean coasts of northwest Venezuela and northern Colombia. They can hook up anytime with ghosts of loved ones who inhabit the *Guajira* Peninsula. Better yet, they can hook up with potential mates at the fertility dance, *Chichimaya.*

As soon as they hit their teens, *Wayuu* girls are hidden away for months, especially from teenage boys. After they are "mature," they can join a *Chichimaya* dancing bash. Boys dance wildly in circles, waving their hats and teasing the girls to chase them. When a girl spots a guy she thinks is hot, she dances after him. If she can trip him and he goes down, he has a hope of marrying her, knowing they'll have sizzling hot sex for the rest of their days.

If he does fall for her and she accepts him, he'll pay her family with a fine dowry of goats. Later, if his wife takes a lover, her family has to return the goats. If hubby plays around: more goats to the in-laws.

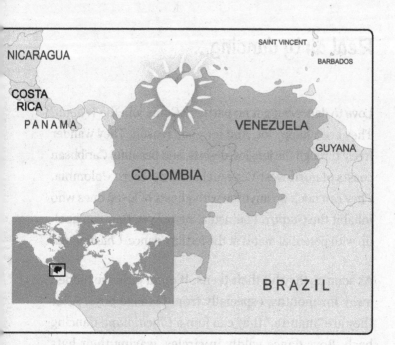

WAYUU OF VENEZUELA AND COLOMBIA

Keep those wholesome family traditions

On the long, lovely beaches of the Trobriand Islands, with its azure waters and coconut palms, life is peaceful and simple. Men fish and grow yams. Women garden and weave skirts. Teenage boys learn ancestral dance and live in a bachelor pad. Teenage girls have sex with any bachelors they choose—variety is the spice of life! Doting parents give their daughters thoughtful advice, such as which boys look like good lovers.

There are rules of propriety, of course. Screwing a guy is fine, but don't you dare engage in a premarital meal. Want to be the village bad girl? Have dinner with a guy before you're married.

Big losers in the Trobriand Islands are the birth control merchants. Trobrianders know that sex doesn't make babies. The proof? They have lots of the former, but few of the latter. Forget the silly notion that intercourse makes women pregnant. It's obvious that the ancestors' spirits (called *baloma*) make women pregnant. Trobrianders acknowledge, though, that intercourse might make her more susceptible to the *baloma*.

All these affairs are not just fun and games. They give couples a chance to test their sexual (and other) compatibility. Young women check out the guys' potential as husbands...and they diligently conduct as much research as possible.

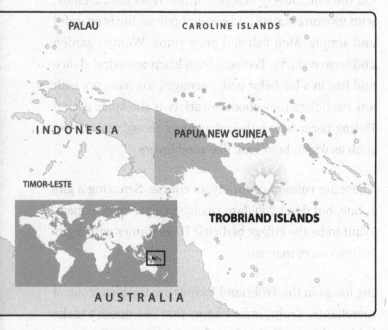

TROBRIAND ISLANDS, PAPUA NEW GUINEA

TERMS OF ENDEARMENT

Tired of trite nicknames for your lover, like "Honey" or "Sweetheart" or "Sugar"? Rev up your romance with these awesome international terms of endearment.

Petit chou (French) – Little cabbage. When your French lover calls you a head of cabbage, he's being romantic, not pushing for an early dinner.

Tamago gata no kao 卵形顔 (Japanese) – Egg with eyes. If your Japanese lover calls you an "egg with eyes," he's flattering your beauty, not commenting on your IQ.

Chuchuzinho (Portugese/Brazil) – Little pumpkin. Your Brazilian lover is being affectionate, not criticizing your figure.

Ma puce (French) – My flea or louse. Your French sweetie is being loving, not complaining that you're as irritating as a flea or head lice.

Chang noi (Thai) – Little elephant. You can use this affectionately to your children, not your husband or lover. Unless, of course, you want to say that his equipment is small.

Polpetta (Italian) – Meatball. You know how important food is to Italians. He's saying you're yummy, not round and squishy.

Chényú luòyàn 沉鱼落雁 (Chinese) – Diving fish, swooping geese. Your Chinese lover is saying you're beautiful, not that you look like a fish with the brains of a goose.

Mijn poepie (Dutch) – My little poo or poopie. Yep, meant with love. Not much more to say about this.

Gordo/gorda (Spanish) – Fatty. A term of affection. Not suggesting you join Weight Watchers.

Khanfoussti / Khanfoussi خنفوسي- خنفوسّتي (Maghreb Arabic) – My little bug. Said tenderly. Not implying you bug the hell out of him/her.

Gang-a-ji 강아지 (Korean) – Puppy. Your darling is saying you're cute, not that you're a dog.

Zhū tóu 猪头 (Chinese) – Pig head. Said lovingly. Not a comment on your appearance or eating habits.

Pulcino (Italian) – Little chicken. Yes, another term of love, not a comment on your brain power or annoying, baseless fears.

Krümel (German) – Crumb. Said fondly. Not related to the English "crummy."

Karale (Malayalam) – Liver. Not comparing you to a large, rubbery organ that secretes bile, but to what (they think) is the source of love. Their version of the Italian *cuore mio*.

Manaraki Μ α ν α ρ α κ ι (Greek) – A small lamb being fed to prepare for slaughter. Said with affection. Not preparing you for getting wooed then dumped (though Greeks do have sex more often than anyone else in the world).

Jigaret Udem (Armenian) – "I will eat your liver." No need to run, unless she's approaching with a carving knife.

Xiao qiu yin 小蚯蚓 (Chinese) – Small earthworm. Term of endearment for a woman, not a comment on a man's character or apparatus.

Gomba (Hungarian) – Mushroom. He's being romantic, not saying you live in the dark and smell like poop.

Moosh bokhoradet موش بخوردت (Persian) – "May a mouse eat you." Commenting on your cuteness, not cheesiness.

Microbino mio (Italian) – "My little microbe." She's saying you're adorable, not that you're making her sick.

Zuzuni Ζ ο υ ζ ο υ ν ι (Greek) – Bug. Again with the insect reference. Not sure what's going on with the Europeans' passion for bugs.

Mijn Bolleke (Flemish) – "My little round thing." Said fondly, not a comment on your hips.

Brzydalu (Polish) – "Ugly one." Hard to figure this one. Maybe follows that old song, "if you want to be happy for the rest of your life, never make a pretty woman your wife…" Except you use it for your man.

Mae-yod-choo (Thai) – "Mother with the most lovers." To be said lovingly by a man to his wife. Implications as you wish.

Looking for a few good men!

The "Sacred Band" was the most famous, powerful, and feared military troop of ancient Greece. These mighty soldiers crushed every foe. They even fought huge legions of the feared Spartans—and won.

The secret of their bravery and military prowess? Their loving, gay relationships. The entire Sacred Band was three hundred carefully chosen male lovers. These guys had unparalleled courage and determination to fight to the death for one another. Of course, they also trained like crazy—mainly dancing and wrestling.

For decades, everyone considered them invincible. That rep only ended when Alexander the Great, of Macedonia, and his dad, King Philip II, defeated all the Greek armies. When King Philip saw the entire Sacred Band lying dead after the battle, he burst into tears. These men, he declared, were the most honorable, bold, and courageous soldiers he had ever fought.

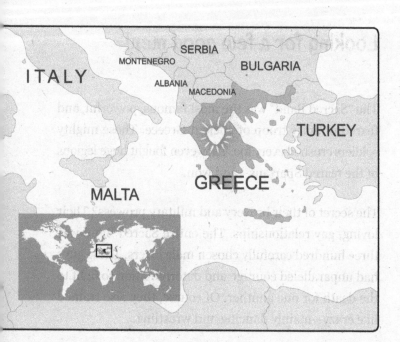

SACRED BAND OF GREECE

Girls just wanna have fun!

Pity the parents of the average teenage girl. Desperate to protect her virginity, they set curfews, declare dress codes, screen boyfriends, chaperone parties.

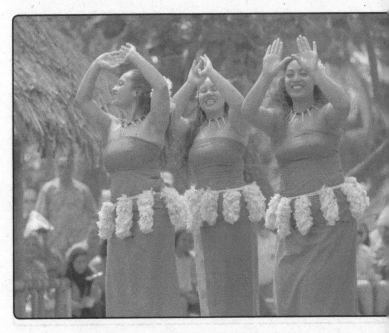

SAMOAN WOMEN TRADITIONAL DANCE

Yet in the innocent days before AIDS, many traditional societies—Bhuiya, Guana, Guaycuru, Kumbi, Akamba, Igorot, Samoan and others—figured teenagers *need* sex.

Take Samoa. Sure, a Samoan girl should learn to cook and weave so she can help support her family. But keep your priorities straight. Tell her to be more responsible and she would protest, "I am but young." The adults understood. When they hit late teens, girls should devote themselves to age-appropriate activities, like having lots of sexual affairs.

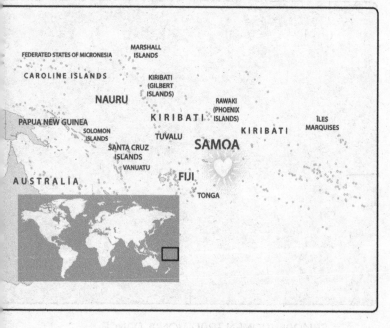

SAMOA

Men are from Venus, Women are from Mars...

"Stick to traditional roles," say the Tchambuli of Papua New Guinea. Men should do what they do best: dance, paint, play the flute. In their villages along Chambri Lake, rich in rare birds and infested with crocodiles, Tchambuli women know what they want—and go after it. *They* are the sexual aggressor and *they* decide whom they'll mate.

To entice the women, Tchambuli men compete constantly, trying out new hairdos and decorating themselves with flowers and ornaments. At Tchambuli festivals, young men dress up as women so they can join in the raunchy homosexual dancing and sex play women enjoy at every festival.

The Tchambuli women are busy with "women's work." They shave their heads and hunt.

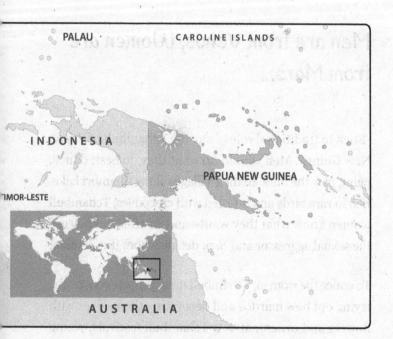

TCHAMBULI OF PAPUA NEW GUINEA

DANGEROUS WEAPONS OUTLAWED

You've got to love this.

Some US states consider dildos dangerous weapons. For example, it's illegal to own a dildo in Sandy Springs, Georgia. Guns are just fine, though. In GA, you can carry guns in your car and bring them into bars. You can bring them to school classrooms, as long as you're dropping off or picking up a student. And you can carry your trusty sidearm into church with the minister's blessing, and into airport TSA safety checkpoints if you have a gun permit. Indeed, in Kennesaw, GA, every homeowner must own a firearm and ammunition (unless they're too poor or too insane).

In Alabama, it's illegal to sell anything you might use to have an orgasm, or as they so quaintly put it: any device "designed or marketed as useful primarily for the stimulation of human genital organs."

In Texas, that bastion of liberty, it was illegal to own more than six dildos until 2008. Then they came to their senses.

No such luck for the upright citizens of Arizona. More than two dildos in the same house can land you in jail.

Sex scrooges need not apply...

The Aché of eastern Paraguay believe the most important human trait is to be a "good giver." They share everything with one another—food, houses, chores, childcare, spouses. Skilled and savvy hunters and foragers, the Aché have roamed thousands of acres of forest over the centuries, from the spectacular *Guairá* waterfalls, south along the *Cordillera de San Rafael* mountains and the *Paraná* River. Wherever they go, they make sure that everyone gets a share of the meal. Afterwards, the women make sure that all the men they like get a piece of the pie.

That doesn't mean Aché women don't believe in marriage—they do! *Lots* of marriages! Women choose their own husbands, and most Aché women have had at least a dozen marriages, with short romances sprinkled along the way.

Think that makes it tough to figure out baby's dad? No problem! The Aché believe every baby is a mix of all the lovers mom chose just before and during her pregnancy. Babies are, after all, developed by the application of lots of semen while mom is pregnant. The result: all kids have several fathers—the man she had sex with just before pregnancy, the man she thinks is responsible for getting her pregnant, any men who donated food while she was pregnant, and her husband.

So no one worries if mom disappears for a week. She'll be home soon...with another dad!

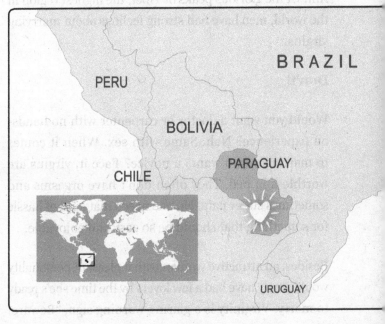

ACHÉ OF PARAGUAY

"Position open. Experience preferred..."

Amidst the glorious peaks of Tibet, the highest region in the world, men have had strong feelings about marrying virgins.

Don't!

Would you want a doctor or carpenter with no hands-on experience? Nah. Same with sex. When it comes to marriage, who wants a novice? Face it, virgins are worthless in bed. They often don't have orgasms and sometimes suffer pain. No one needs that kind of hassle for something that should be so easy and enjoyable.

Besides, an attractive woman with a pleasant personality would surely have had a few lovers by the time she's ready to marry. Virginity is a glaring warning sign, "Beware! There's something wrong with her." If you absolutely must make love to a virgin, at least don't marry her. Be smart and wait until she's had a little practice.

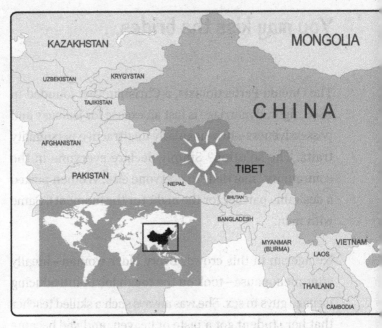

TIBET AUTONOMOUS REGION OF CHINA

You may kiss the brides...

The Oneida Perfectionists, a Christian sect founded in 1848, figured marriage is just an excuse for jealousy and possessiveness—two singularly unattractive personality traits. The solution? Simply declare everyone in the community "married" to everyone else. Women picked a desirable partner for the night (or the moment). Same with men.

No ageism in this crowd. Every older woman—ideally after menopause—took on the tough job of introducing teenage guys to sex. She was always such a skilled teacher that her student got a taste of heaven, and she became his religious role model.

Must be all that practice.

No slouches, elderly men were always willing to step up and do their duty teaching late-teen gals.

The founder of the Oneida community, John Noyes, also introduced *stirpiculture*, selective breeding. Sure, all adults could have sex with all other adults. But only some of that bumping and grinding should produce offspring. If you wanted kids, you had to apply for the privilege. If you had spiritual superiority, Noyes and his committee matched you with the right breeding partner. Magically, Noyes himself passed the test so often he fathered 20 percent of the kids born in the community.

Alas, this utopia didn't last. Noyes absconded to Canada to avoid arrest in New York. The other members peeled away over time. But the Oneida community didn't die; it just faded into a corporation, Oneida Silverware, still one of the world's largest silverware manufacturers.

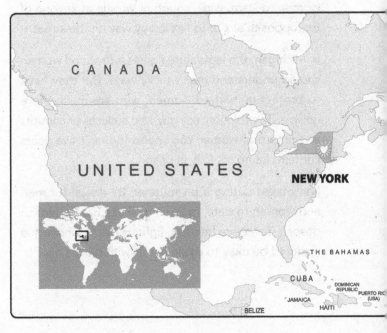

ONEIDA COMMUNITY OF NEW YORK, USA

DATE NIGHT... NOT!

It wasn't so long ago that dating was forbidden virtually everywhere. Ah, how times have changed...or not.

Forget Sadie Hawkins Day if you live in Dyersburg, Tennessee. It's illegal for a woman to call a man for a date.

The legislators of Little Rock, Arkansas, are dedicated to protecting people from flirts. It's illegal for men or women to stare, wink, cough or whistle at anyone of the opposite sex or to flirt in any way on the street.

In Michigan, the legislature figures a divorced woman should understand men's tricky ways. But they have to protect unmarried women, who are much more gullible. The solution: any guy who seduces or corrupts an unmarried woman can spend the next five years contemplating his folly in prison.

Iran makes dating a bit tougher. It's illegal for men and women to date, or even to shake hands. Not to despair. There are freedom-fighters in Iran who argue it should be okay to shake hands with gloves on.

Junk Match.com!

Hot for a guy who's oblivious to your charms? The Nenet women of Siberia can help! In the frozen tundra, Nenet women have adapted skillfully to the harsh environment. They make clothes that protect from -40°F winters, slit open reindeer so everyone can gobble raw liver, kidney, lungs, and heart, and can pack up the whole household tent in a flash, even in a blizzard.

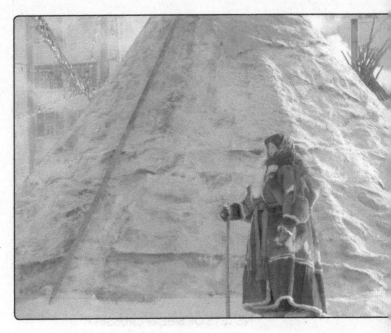

NENET WOMAN STANDING BEFORE HER TENT

Every Nenet woman is also savvy about snaring a reluctant lover. She easily imposes complete and total control over him. She can even use magical commands to rule his every thought and action.

How does she seize this bewitching power? Easy! She simply steps over any possession he has left on the ground—and he's her pawn for life.

That'll teach him to pick up his socks.

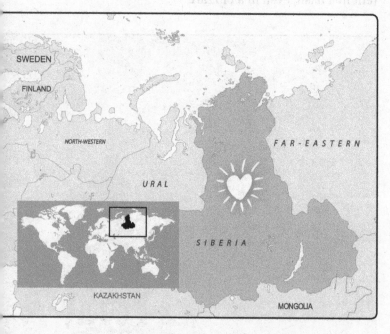

NENETS OF SIBERIA, RUSSIA

Obey your elders!

Better yet, take them to bed, say the Apanyekrá-Canela of Brazil. The Canela villages of the savanna, with tropical forests and streams, are rich in fish and game. The sex lives of young Canela men are just as rich. All young men in their mid-to-late teens get initiated into sex by "experienced" young women. After that first delight, every young man spends several years in training, having sex only with women at least thirty years older than he is.

The Canela say sex between young people—even married couples—is unhealthy. Horny young guys should get it on with women in their late forties or fifties. Sex with older women will make him strong and courageous, while sex with a younger woman—even his wife—will make him weak and nervous.

Any man who strays and has sex with a young woman is shamed and hazed before the whole village. He has to walk down a line of dancing women, all laughing and teasing him.

And for you horny young gals? Patience, honey. Best wait until you're older. On the other hand, if you do break the rules, everyone will pretty much ignore it.

While a guy gets educated by the Golden Girls, his parents choose a fiancée for him. As soon as she's old enough to have sex with him, the two decide whether to get married or split up. If she likes him, her family buys him from his family with a large meat pie. The meat pie seals the deal. Afterwards, if he wants out, his family must pay her family a heavy fine. But if she wants out, it's just *sayonara, baby*.

Made a mistake and now stuck in a sorry marriage? Either spouse can easily initiate divorce—as long as they have no kids.

Once a woman is pregnant, the whole deal changes. Women continue to be free to end the marriage any time, and if she throws him out, he must leave immediately. For husbands, though, it's tough luck. If he initiates divorce, his family and friends totally harass him, and he must pay a hefty fine.

This is fair because "real" men are reasonable, non-competitive, and totally cooperative. Only animals and women get into outright conflict. When a woman is irritable, irrational, demanding, or fickle, her husband's job is to quietly appease her. If she plays around, it's certainly not grounds for divorce or even raised voices. But if he comes home and she's in their bed with another man, the guy should at least give him a gift.

Sex, Lies and Virgins' Tastes or How to Pick a Lover

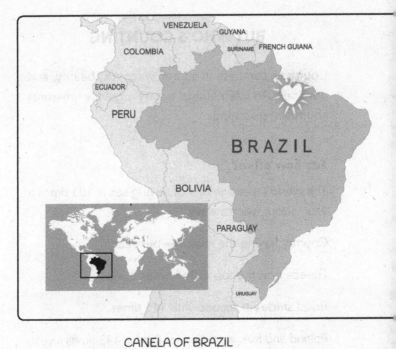

CANELA OF BRAZIL

BUT WHO'S COUNTING

Countries compete in sports, weapons, beauty, and now, sex. An international survey regularly measures countries' sex ratings.

Sex how often?

The world's average rate of having sex is 103 times a year, about twice a week.

Country having the most sex per year?

Greece is at the top at 164 times a year.

Brazil strides in second with 145 times.

Poland and Russia are tied for third at 143 times a year.

Least often?

Japan, at forty-eight times per year.

Of course, maybe the Japanese just answered more honestly than other countries.

How good?

The average satisfaction with their sexual experience, worldwide — 43%. Alas, not quite half of us enjoy getting it on.

The countries most satisfied with their sex lives?

#1 is Nigeria! Where 67% say they are very satisfied.

Mexico is second with 63% very satisfied.

India comes in third with 61% very satisfied.

The USA, by the way, at 48%, is only slightly higher than the average. That's behind Mexico 63%, India 61%, Poland 54%, Greece 51%, Holland 50%, South Africa 50%, and Spain 49%.

Maybe that's why 46% of US women surveyed said, if they have to give up something for two weeks, they'd rather give up sex than the Internet.

Least sexually satisfied country?

Japan, with only 15% satisfied. Of course, we all know the Japanese have higher standards.

Just a few salt grains to toss on these results. Nigeria was the only country that took the survey face to face instead of online. Imagine sitting next to your main squeeze. The surveyor asks how satisfied you are with the sex. Do you say, "Ehh, not so much"?

Spain apparently wasn't thrilled with the results, so they did their own survey. It showed that 90% were sexually satisfied. Go figure.

The Italians also dissed the survey, which showed a paltry 36% satisfied. In a different "sex of the nations survey," 64% of Italians said they were satisfied with their sex lives.

How long?

Surveys show that the length of intercourse directly affects satisfaction.

Longest intercourse?

The Nigerians again top the charts at 24 minutes per session.

Shortest?

Indians, at 13 minutes. Maybe the Indians can devote another 10 minutes and get their satisfaction rate up.

What's love got to do with it?

It seems all the world is romantic. Ninety-six percent of both women and men say sex is better when there's an emotional connection.

How early?

The average age of first having sex, worldwide? Eighteen-and-a-half.

Early birds?

Iceland at fifteen-and-a-half. Great way to stay warm.

Latest to indulge?

Malaysia at age twenty-three.

Ditch the steroids...

Try semen instead, say the Etoro of the central mountains in Papua New Guinea. Way healthier and more effective.

Is homosexuality unnatural or healthy?
Proper or offensive?

The Etoro have no doubt. *All* men should have a male lover.

But no sense being an extremist. "Go ahead," urge the Etoro, "marry—even have sex with your wife. Just realize it will kill you."

Want to scandalize your Etoro neighbors? Totally gross them out with something really disgusting? Probably get banished?

Have sex with your wife in your house.

Everyone knows the only decent place to have sex with a spouse is in the forest.

In their villages along the lower slopes of the extinct volcano Mt. Sisa, the Etoro hunt and garden, and avoid acts that drain their life force. They ban sex between men and women for eight months a year. Sex between men and women is **always** taboo in or near houses or vegetable gardens.

Homosexual oral sex is another story—perfectly fine anytime, anywhere, because it makes crops thrive and young men strong.

Want *The Force* to be with you? Grow vigorous and powerful? Drink plenty of semen. Each Etoro young man selects a male partner who helps ensure he gets his daily semen ration.

Women, on the other hand, tend to "waste" semen by often having sex without getting pregnant.

As you might guess, the Etoro pose no threat of over-population.

How come some societies ban homosexuality and others promote it? Some social scientists say it's all about food: where food shortages are common, people tend to accept homosexuality. Plenty of food, lots more homophobia.

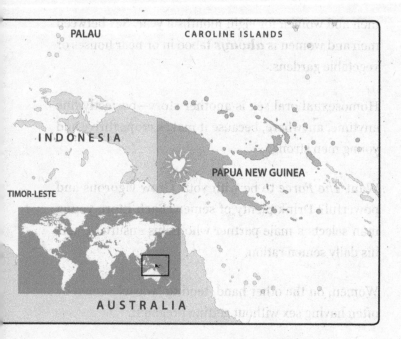

ETORO OF PAPUA NEW GUINEA

Make love...and war

Legend says the Amazons were brutal, courageous warrior-women. Scoffers claim they are only a myth. But who are you going to believe, Herodotus or a bunch of kill-joys?

Herodotus, "father of history" in the fifth century BC, reported on the Amazons. He said these awesome women battled and pillaged for thousands of miles. They also got high on cannabis, built saunas, and had lots of tattoos.

Once a year, they hooked up with some local deserving tribe to party and get pregnant. They sent the resulting baby boys back to their dads, and kept the girls to follow in mom's footsteps and become great warriors.

Though they could crush any foes in combat, they eventually capitulated to love. They met the Scythians on the battlefield—some seriously powerful dudes themselves. As the two sides got ready to fight, they thought each other was smokin'. Instead of cutting out the enemies' hearts, the Amazons decided to surrender their own. The two sides gave up battling each other for pillaging together.

Their descendants kept mom's family traditions. They created a society of nomads where women and men were equals. The women hunted on horseback, fought as soldiers alongside the men, and refused to marry until they had killed a man in battle.

Until the 1990s, most historians thought the Amazons were just a crazed fantasy. Then archaeologists discovered graves of warrior women that proved the Amazon stories. These were super-women—5'6" tall—amazingly tall for the time. They wore pants, had tattoos, were bowlegged from constant riding, and got buried with their weapons and pot paraphernalia. They created the free lives they wanted and could hold their own in love or war with any man.

Wonder Woman Lives!

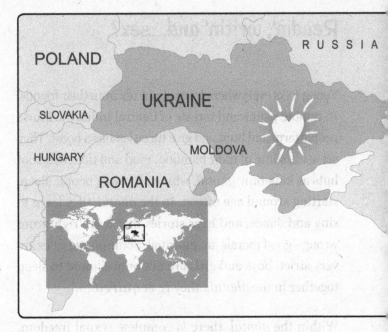

AMAZONS (UKRAINE)

Readin', writin' and...sex?

Young folks everywhere learn about sex from their friends. In remote plains and forests of Central India, the Muria people farm and hunt and give those lessons a boost. They set aside some of their bamboo, mud and thatched-roof huts as kids-only *ghotul*, where all young people sleep, starting around age fifteen. In the *ghotul*, they learn to sing and dance, and hear stories that teach right from wrong—good morals are essential. Some *ghotul* rules are very strict: boys and girls are not only allowed to sleep together in the *ghotul*...they're **required** to.

Within the *ghotal,* there is complete sexual freedom. Teens who like each other can indulge in sex to their hearts' content. The golden rule is that practice makes perfect, and plenty of intercourse helps them refine their skills in the sexual arts. The only rule for kids: switch partners often. No one should feel left out.

The rule for adults: *Keep out!*

The Muria also forbid child marriage and think it's barbaric.

If two young adults decide to marry, they must separate immediately after the wedding and wait an entire year before they meet again. When the year is over, if they're still mutually charmed, they are reunited forever...or until wife or husband decides to change spouses.

Think the *ghotul* a little too risqué? Consider the evidence. Divorce rates in the West hover near 50 percent. Among the Muria? Less than 4 percent. Until the Muria started socializing with outsiders a few years ago, sexually transmitted diseases were rare and HIV/AIDS nonexistent.

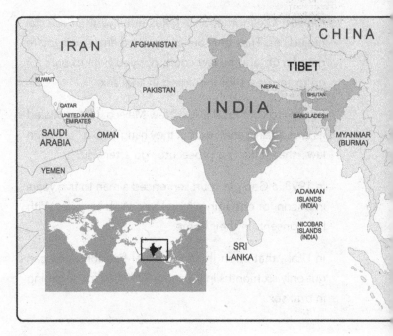

MURIA OF INDIA

FOR MISSIONARIES ONLY

Enjoy sex that's not the missionary position? Better avoid some parts of the USA.

In Washington, DC, the only acceptable sexual position is missionary-style. Anything else is illegal.

Alabama, Florida, Idaho, Michigan, Mississippi, North Carolina, South Carolina, and Utah all have laws that outlaw oral and/or anal sex between any consenting adults.

Kansas, Oklahoma, and Texas indulge their special prejudices. They only outlaw oral and anal sex if you're gay. An Oklahoma law could put you behind bars for up to ten years for indulging in anal sex.

Be nice to your local DA in New Mexico. NM repealed its laws against anal sex, but they hang onto a "common law" that still lets a prosecutor go after you.

In 1998, a Georgia court sentenced a man to five years in prison for engaging in oral sex. With his wife. With her consent. In their home.

In Utah, that stronghold of sexual freedom, you can get only six months in jail and a $299 fine for engaging in oral sex.

It's worth noting that the US Supreme Court declared all these laws unconstitutional in 2003, so legislatures that passed them are breaking the highest law in the land.

A boy and his soa...

Surrounded by towering waterfalls, stunning golden beaches and clear, turquoise waters, Samoan kids are more outgoing, warm, and friendly than kids in most other countries. A Samoan boy likes to do *everything* with his best friend, his *soa*—play together, do chores together, get circumcised together.

He also counts on his *soa* to score a girlfriend for him— he can't possibly pursue her himself. *Wa-a-a-y* too embarrassing. He sends his *soa* to sing his praises and convince his chosen sweetheart that he's a great catch. But the wise boy chooses his *soa* very carefully. A *soa* who is too cool and fine might end up winning her for himself.

A boy with a paranoid streak recruits several *soa* at the same time, and sends them out to eavesdrop on each other. He just keeps fingers crossed that they don't all turn out to be traitors.

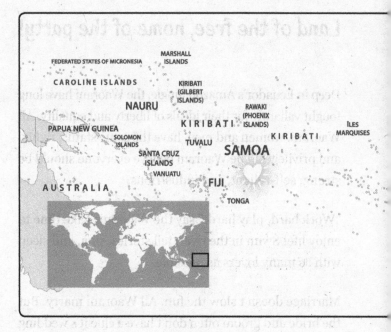

SAMOA

Land of the free, home of the party!

Deep in Ecuador's Amazon jungle, the Waorani have long fought valiantly for their ideals of liberty and equality. All Waorani, women and men, have the same status, rights, and privileges. The Waorani believe everyone should be strong, self-reliant, and industrious.

"Work hard, play hard!" say the Waorani. Take time to enjoy life! Swim in the river, tell stories, sing, and sleep with as many lovers as possible.

Marriage doesn't slow the fun. All Waorani marry. But the bride and groom often don't have a clue it's wedding day. During a drinking festival, older relatives sit the unwitting couple together in a hammock, sing a little song over them. Then...

Surprise! You're hitched!

No worries. You're always free to dump the spouse. Most couples stay together, though, because marriage helps you live well. The idea of romantically "falling in love" is silly. But spouses are fond and respectful of one another. Besides, it's not as though you're stuck as just a twosome. An active sex life with many people before and during marriage is healthy and normal. Multiple wives or husbands? Sure. All it takes is a swing in a hammock and you've tied the knot.

It's also important to be practical. Once a woman is pregnant, she needs to take several lovers who will all contribute the semen needed to create the child. That way, the babe has a safety net—several fathers to watch over her, in case one or more dies or leaves.

Sex with the same gender? Why not? Whatever works for both parties is up to them.

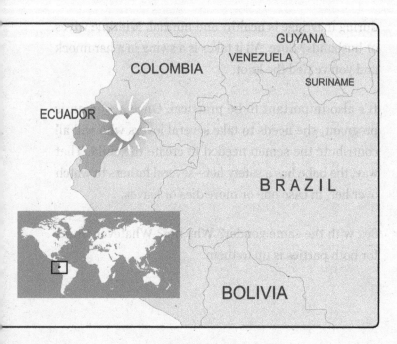

WAORANI OF ECUADOR

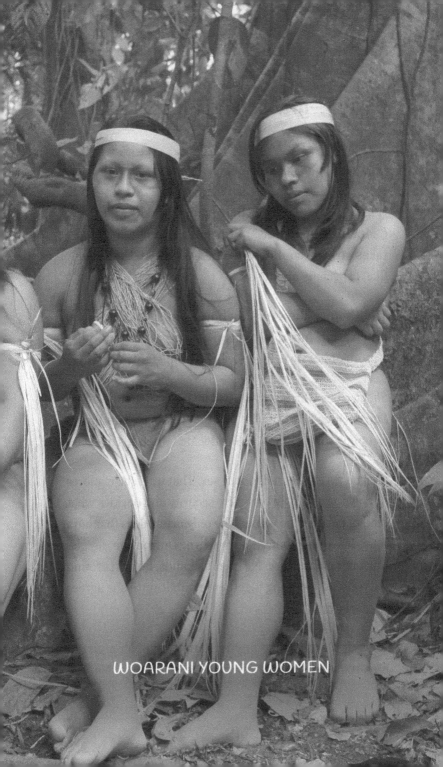

WOARANI YOUNG WOMEN

Crotch-grabbers get lost!

Want a happy, passionate marriage?

"Easy!" say the Kreung of the beautiful, remote *Ratanakiri* ("Mountain of Jewels") Province in Cambodia. It just takes strong, confident women who know what they like, especially about sex.

The Kreung know exactly how to raise such women. When a girl hits mid-teens, Kreung parents build her a room of her own. There, she's completely in charge.

She decides which boy she will invite to spend the night. *She* decides how they'll spend it. Talking... cuddling... sleeping...or having sex. *She* decides when it's over.

She makes all the rules about sex. That way, she explores her own sexuality in complete security and decides what kind of partner she wants. The only firm rule is that boys must leave her room before dawn. During the day, he must not go near her. No holding hands, no arm around the waist, no walking together in public until she agrees to marry him.

Boys don't dare take any initiative, or push a girl to do any more than she offers. When she says, "No," he obeys immediately and without question. The penalties for anything else would be severe, for both him and his parents.

Can't beat the stats. Divorce among the Krueng is extremely rare. Rape and sexual assault are virtually nonexistent.

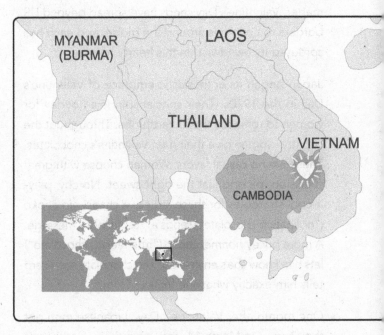

KREUNG OF CAMBODIA

VALENTINE'S DAY
AROUND THE WORLD

Since concocted in 1700s USA, Valentine's Day is the celebration of love and romance. Of course cynics suspect its popularity might be tied to the $18 billion total price tag for all that candy, cards, and flowers. No matter: Valentine's Day seeds have spread beyond US borders to countries around the globe, and each has sprouted its own twist on this hearty holiday.

Japan began its enthusiastic embrace of Valentine's Day in the 1970s. Their special spin is a holiday for women to romance their heartthrobs. Throughout the country, women give their men Valentine's chocolates. These are no casual favors. Women choose with great precision, picking just the right sweet. No coy, play-it-cool strategies for these ladies. A cheap *giri choko* ("obligation chocolate") sends a "just friends" message. A more pricey *honmei choko* ("true feeling chocolate") lets him know she's enamored. The chocolate scorecard tells him exactly what she thinks of him.

One month after Valentine's Day, Japanese men get their turn. On March 14, they give their sweethearts "White Day" white chocolates, white flowers, or other small gifts.

Like Japan, South Korean Valentine's is the day women give their men chocolates. And like Japan, Korean men do their part a month later. But the Koreans are an empathetic bunch, and think those without sweethearts need a special day too. Enter April 14, "Black Day." Didn't give or get a Valentine in February and March? You get your chance in April. On the 14th, join your other single friends for a dinner date of *jajangmyeon* (black bean-paste noodles).

The Chinese Valentine's Day is the *Qixi* (Double Seventh) Festival, held on the seventh day of the seventh month on the Chinese calendar (August 28 in 2017). It celebrates the annual reuniting of star-crossed lovers. A more cheery Romeo and Juliet – instead of dying, they simply re-connect once a year.

In Spain, Catalonians have their own version of Valentine's Day, called Saint Jordi day, April 23. Romantic women give books to the men in their lives. Men give women roses. Like good capitalists everywhere, enterprising vendors set up book-and-flower stalls around Barcelona. The government also obliges by opening the Government Palace to visitors on Saint Jordi Day, where people watch the blessing of the roses in the Palace's Gothic courtyard. Some say the holiday also has roots in the myth of St. George (Saint Jordi), who slayed a dragon to save a princess and a city.

Ever the romantics, Russian men give chocolates and presents to their special women on International Women's Day. In case you have been living in a cave without women, International Women's Day, March 8, celebrates women's economic and political achievements. It highlights political and social awareness of the struggles of women worldwide.

In the Philippines, people take *Araw ng mga Puso* (Valentine's Day) in a different direction – straight to the marriage ceremony. Filipinos love things big – big families, big parties, and now, big Valentine's Day events. Thousands gather on February 14th to participate in a mass wedding, usually held free in Manila. Even more like to celebrate the day with a kissing festival. On Valentine's Day 2004, in Manila, 5,300 couples simultaneously kissed for ten seconds, breaking the world record.

Argentinians got the message that Valentine's Day is a great revenue-generator. Argentina, home of the tango, one of the world's sexiest dances, has the world's longest "celebration of love." During Sweetness Week in July, lovers exchange candy and kisses for seven days.

What's love without competition? On Valentine's Day in 2013, a Thai couple set the record for the world's longest kiss: 58 hours, 35 minutes and 58 seconds.

Nine couples entered the contest, including a married couple in their seventies.

The Danes figure love means you can take a joke. On Valentine's Day, they send joke cards. One can imagine:

> Roses are red,
> Violets are blue,
> I might be in love,
> But not with you

Germans like Valentines with that cuddly animal that clearly symbolizes love and passion, the pig. So if your German lover calls you a pig, don't be hurt. It's a romantic term of undying love. Not too surprising in the land of beer and sausages.

In 2015, the Indian Hindu nationalist party Mahasabha decided lovers' actions should speak louder than words. They looked for unsuspecting couples out on Valentine's Day, and strongly urged them to get married. Right now! No use trying to procrastinate. They had religious leaders on call to marry them immediately.

World's most romantic country?

Which is the world's most romantic country? France, with Paris, the city of lights and love? Or Italy, with the canals and gondolas of Venice? Maybe the Philippines—home of the world's largest Valentine's Day mass wedding?

Ah, but they all pale beside diligently romantic Republic of Korea, where they celebrate a "Love Day" on the fourteenth of *every month of the year*:

January 14 – Diary Day. Give your beloved a blank diary, presumably to record the endearing moments you will share.

February 14 – Valentine's Day. Women, give your guys chocolates.

March 14 – White Day. Guys, you get to return the Valentine's Day favor with white chocolates, white flowers, or presents. Just be sure your gift costs about three times the one you got from her in February.

April 14 – Black Day. A love time for singles to commiserate—or celebrate—with other single friends over a bowl of black bean noodles.

May 14 – Yellow Day. Dress in yellow, along with your better half, and exchange yellow roses. Single? You can eat yellow curry to encourage the love spirits to spice up your life with a new lover.

June 14 – Kiss Day. What else? The day to pucker up with your smooch-mate. Better yet, lay one on someone you'd like to fall in love with.

July 14 – Silver Day. Time to get serious. Exchange silver "promise" rings with your lover and start making wedding plans.

August 14 – Green Day. After all that talk of weddings, you need Green Day, dedicated to drinking rice vodka (*soju*). Down enough and you can stumble through a romantic walk in green woods with your beloved.

September 14 – Photo Day. When are Koreans *not* taking photos? Never mind. Today is "official" photo day. Time to click a few candids with your *jagiya* (sweetie).

October 14 – Wine Day. Spring for a nice bottle of vino for your honey. Single? Oh well, more for you.

November 14 – Movie Day. Hit the theatres, rent some DVDs, or go to a Korean "DVD Bang," where you hang out with your pals, make out with your SO, and watch romantic movies.

December 14 – Hug Day. Pre-empt the New Year with a big one for your main squeeze. You also get to vote for the celebrity who is most huggable.

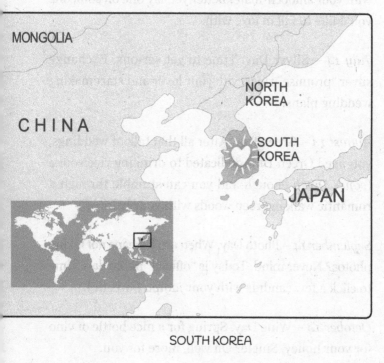

MONGOLIA

CHINA

NORTH KOREA

SOUTH KOREA

JAPAN

SOUTH KOREA

THE VALENTINE'S GRINCH

Who could object to love and romance, hearts and flowers, chocolates and lace? Apparently, lots of people. In some countries, give a Valentine, get a jail sentence.

Saudi Arabia's religious police outlawed anything that smacked of Valentine's Day. You can get arrested for the criminal act of buying anything that suggests Valentine's Day in any way. Women wearing red. Merchants selling any red object. Anyone buying candy with red wrapping. Indeed, in 2012, they arrested 140 people for those heinous deeds. In 2014, five Saudis got a total, between them, of thirty-nine years behind bars and 4,500 cane lashes for the crime of dancing with unmarried women on Valentine's Day.

Iran's "morality" police also aim to ensure no one publicly celebrates Valentine's Day. They close down any shop that is reckless (or romantic) enough to sell anything decorated with hearts and flowers around V-day.

Malaysia's Islamic authorities have forbidden Muslims from celebrating Valentine's Day. In 2014, the Islamic morality police (JAIS) arrested eighty Muslim couples for celebrating Valentine's Day.

Indonesians are generally as romantic as anyone — but not in the province of Aceh. They banned the day of flowers and candy for lovers, and warned they were not fooling around. A major association of Aceh religious scholars said there'd be severe punishment for anyone caught surreptitiously celebrating Valentine's Day.

Not just another pretty face...

Each year, the Wodaabe nomads drive their cattle hundreds of miles—from southern Niger, through northern Nigeria and Cameroon, to southwestern Chad and sometimes beyond—to seek grazing land along the edges of the Sahara desert. The Wodaabe are known for their modesty, patience, generosity, loyalty, and good looks. They celebrate their beauty with the *Guérewol*, the annual beauty pageant...for men.

Hey, guys, want to be a contestant? Clear your calendar. This will take days. First, shave your hairline way back. Then smooth a layer of red clay all over your face. Carefully apply thick black eyeliner and black lip paint. Draw a white line straight down the center of your nose so it will look as long as possible. Slip into your finest embroidered tunic, pop on your headdress of ostrich feathers and horsehair.

Then dance in a long line of men for the *Yaake* dance competition, as temps climb to 104°F. Vibrate your throat, lips and mouth, roll your eyes to show how white they are, flash those pearly teeth, while stretching on tiptoes into the air like a bird. It's all to score points with the women judges.

The fun isn't over yet. For the rest of the week, you'll dance in the *Guérewol* competition, where young women judge your beauty and skills to decide if you're marriage or lover material.

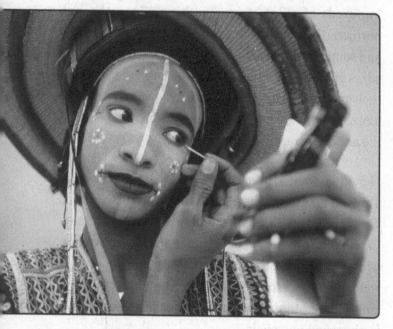

WODAABE MAN AT GUÉREWOL CONTEST

With all that male beauty fluttering around, no wonder unmarried Wodaabe women are free to have sex with anyone they wish. Married women are more staid—they can simply marry more than one gorgeous dude.

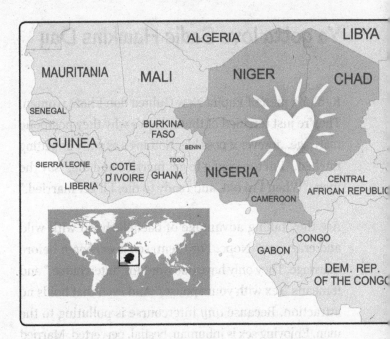

WODAABE OF NIGER, NIGERIA, CAMEROON, CHAD

Ya gotta love Sadie Hawkins Day

Kaulong men of Papua New Guinea don't hate women. They're just terrified of them. That's why they postpone marriage...forever if possible. Nothing's as scary as getting hitched. "I'm too young to get married and die," say the men. "When I'm old, and ready to die, I'll get married."

Are they taking advantage of bachelorhood with wild and crazy sex? Nope. For them, sex is *verboten* before marriage. They only have one word for "intercourse," and it means "sex with your spouse." And even that holds no attraction. Because *any* intercourse is polluting to the man. Enjoying sex is inhuman, bestial, perverted. Married couples who spend time alone, away from the group, are sick with a disgusting animal obsession with sex.

Women figure it differently. When her guy flees from sex, she's the aggressor. She starts with something simple. Cook a few tidbits of food spiced with magical potions to destroy her intended's will to flee. Add a little flirting. Top it off with an attack using whips and knives.

He can run like hell or, if he's smitten, stand his ground and offer some gifts in return. But if he surrenders to her seductions, he's guilty of rape. Then he takes his choice: marriage or death.

If he initiates *any* act of courtship—evil stuff like bringing her flowers—he's guilty of rape. In the good old days, she would decide whether to marry him or have him executed. Things are a bit more lenient these days.

Women can marry late, or not at all—her choice. If she finds some guy enticing, her brothers and sisters will capture the reluctant groom and hold him hostage until he accepts his marital fate.

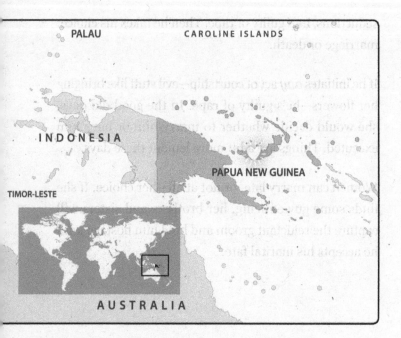

KAULONG OF PAPUA NEW GUINEA

THE M WORD

Masturbation is one of those rare things that feels good and is also good for you. Despite its obvious benefits, many places want to deny its citizens this wholesome activity.

First the good. Masturbation goes way back. A clay figurine of a woman masturbating dates back to the fourth millennium BC. And no wonder. Masturbation is cheap, easy, and offers a wide range of physical, mental, and sexual health benefits.

Take the psychological benefits. There's improved sense of well-being, which should be of interest to anyone. Higher self-esteem and better body image – good for those who are taller, shorter, fatter, thinner, or whatever, than they wish. It lowers stress – great for businesspeople and moms everywhere. It reduces depression – helpful to anyone who believes in climate change.

Masturbation also brings many physical benefits. Better sleep, lower muscle tension, lower risk of type-2 diabetes. Orgasms from masturbation can even strengthen your immune system. Just for women: fewer menstrual cramps, fewer cervical infections, and better muscle tone in the pelvic and anal areas, which reduce the chance of involuntary urine leakage and uterine prolapse. For men: lower risk of prostate cancer.

Then there are the sexual health benefits: better sex with a partner, more and better orgasms, reduced sexual dysfunction, greater physical and emotional satisfaction with relationships, lower sexual tension, no chance of getting an STD, and the chance to enjoy sexual pleasure even if you lack a partner.

No wonder almost everybody does it. In a study of Sweden, Belgium and Germany, 95 percent of males and 89 percent of females report that they have ever masturbated. The numbers seem to be similar in the USA. The stats are likely the same in most other countries.

Then the bad. Despite its popularity and many benefits, social stigmas against masturbation persist. They may not stop many people, but they can embarrass them… or worse. Much of this prejudice in the Western world stems from (why are you not surprised) disinformation from ignorant media. It goes all the way back to the sixteenth century. The big push came from a book with the catchy title *Onania, or the Heinous Sin of Self-Pollution, And All Its Frightful Consequences, In Both Sexes, Considered: With Spiritual and Physical Advice To Those Who Have Already Injured Themselves By This Abominable Practice*. The writer argued that masturbation was not only a sin, it actually made you sick, disfigured, and impotent. Like so much of today's fake news, it combined conservative moralistic diatribe with fake "science." And like so much recent fake news, it was hugely successful. Lots of people were convinced of total lies for centuries.

Sadly, enlightenment is slow coming. In 1994, the US Surgeon General Joycelyn Elders was fired because she suggested that high school sex education programs should be able to discuss masturbation. Apparently, the increase of HIV and other STDs and unintended pregnancies is better, according to her critics, than discussing masturbation as a sexual outlet.

And now the ugly. Some governments make laws to withhold this healthy pleasure from its citizens. The state of Michigan, for example, has a law forbidding a man to engage "in acts of gross indecency, either in public or private." This includes the simple act of solitary masturbation. Penalty: up to five years in prison.

Indonesia has made masturbation illegal. Pleasure yourself and you can land in prison for up to thirty-two months.

Worse yet, masturbate in Saudi Arabia and you can get three years in prison and three hundred lashes. Unlike the US states with anti-masturbation laws, the Saudis seem determined to enforce them. In March 2004, a Saudi court sentenced a teacher to three years in prison and three hundred lashes for saying that Islam does not forbid masturbation (as well as homosexuality, smoking, and music).

The "opposite" sex?

In 2016, Oregon made it legal to be neither male nor female, but a third gender. Progressives applauded. Very liberated...only hundreds of years behind many cultures around the world.

Take the Bugis, the largest ethnic group in South Sulawesi, Indonesia. Centuries ago they recognized five genders. Each has its own charms.

There are the *makkunrai*, which some folks today call "cis-women." These are people who are labeled "female" at birth and identify as women.

The second gender is the *oroani*. They would be called "cis-men"—people labeled "male" at birth, who identify as men.

The third gender is the *calalai*. They are labeled "female" at birth but feel and act traditionally masculine. *Calalai* hold "men's" jobs, freely walk alone at night, dress in pants or a men's sarong, and generally seem to fit their society's sense of "masculine." They often live with female partners and adopt children. They are not considered men, nor do they want to be. Why would they? They have way more freedom than ordinary men or women. They proudly say they are *calalai*.

The fourth gender is the *calabai*. They are labeled "male" at birth but feel and act traditionally feminine. *Calabai* are not considered women, either by themselves or others. They are happy to be their own distinct gender, with freedoms forbidden to ordinary men or women. *Calabai* can dress as both women and men. They can fit into both "men's" and "women's" worlds. They also have unique talents. For example, *calabai* are famous for arranging wonderful weddings.

The fifth gender is the *bissu*. They are shamans who transcend any single gender category. You can't just decide to become a *bissu*. You must be born with the *bissu* potential and work hard to fulfill it. The *bissu* harmoniously combine all of the traditionally "male" and "female" traits. Their role is to ensure that all five genders live together in a healthy, peaceful way so that the universe is in harmony.

All this makes it easy to answer that earth-shaking question in the US: which public bathroom can people use? The *bissu*, the *calabai* and the *calalai* are all welcome to enter both the "women's" and the "men's" areas, including bathrooms. *Makkunrai* must stick to the women's rooms. *Oroani,* the men's.

Sure would reduce the hysteria level in some state legislatures.

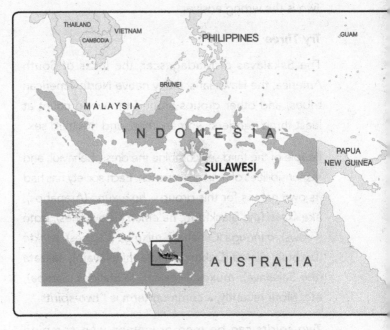

BUGIS OF SOUTH SULAWESI, INDONESIA

HOW MANY GENDERS ARE THERE?

Two is the wrong answer.

Try Three

The Sakalavas of Madagascar, the Incas of South America, the Hawaiians, many native North American tribes, and other groups around the world count at least three genders: women, men, and the third sex.

People of the third sex combine the dress, behavior, and responsibilities of men and women. Each society has had its own names for this group – *hoxuxunó* (Arapahos), *ake:śkassi* (the Blackfoot), *he'eman* (Cheyennes), *boté* (Crows), *minquga* (Omahas), *mixu'ga* (Osages), *winkté* (Lakota), *winkta* (Dakota), *nádleehí* (Navajo), *sekrata* (the Sakalava), *muxes* (Mexico), *fa'afafines* (Samoa), etc. More recently, a common term is "*two-spirits*."

Two-spirits can be men or women who combine traditional male-female characteristics. The physical traits are not important. What counts are the individual's spirit and self-image. They are valuable, high-status members of society, with important social, spiritual, and economic roles. They are known for being clever, hard-working, and generous. Often they can do things that ordinary women and men cannot. In many societies, for example, they are powerful healers. In some, they are the "neutral" judge in disputes between men and women. Imagine how much this saves in divorce lawyer fees.

They also have a knack for mediating between humans and spirits. The gods created *two-spirits* so they'd have someone who could understand them and speak their language. By creating *two-spirits*, they helped all humans improve.

There is just one strong ban about *two-spirits*. Trying to change them. Do that and you bring down disaster on yourself and your society.

Or How About Four?

Lots of folks think four is the right number of genders. Among the Maori, for example, ordinary women and men make up two genders. The third gender is the *whakawahine*, people with male genitals who prefer the company of women and take up traditionally feminine occupations such as weaving. The fourth are *whakatane*, those with female genitals who pursue traditionally male roles, such as becoming a warrior or doing hard physical labor.

Shall We Go for Five?

Four not enough? Try five. Many societies say there are at least five genders. The Navajo, for example, have:

1. *Asdzaan*, meaning woman, is the female gender. It is key in Navajo origin stories, and the most important gender.

2. *Hastiin*, meaning man, is the male gender. It's the other dominant gender, though not as important as woman.

3. *Nadleeh*/hermaphrodite: a third gender, "*nadleeh*," has three forms. One is *nadleeh* that Western medicine calls "hermaphrodite," a person who has both female and male genitals.

4. Female-bodied *nadleeh* (also called *dilbaa*) are people who have female genitals and take the look, work, and roles of men. Traditionally, they have specific ceremonial roles.

5. Male-bodied *nadleeh* are people who have male genitals and take the look, work, and roles of women.

More than Five?

Need more than five? Check out Facebook, which has fifty-plus gender categories to choose from.

None?

Then there are societies that don't have gender categories at all. The Yoruba of Nigeria, for example, don't separate people into male and female. They have no words to distinguish between male and female children or siblings – no words for son, daughter, brother, or sister. The same names are used for girls and boys. The words for husband and wife have nothing to do with gender – you are one or the other depending on your status. Same for rulers. Not "king" and "queen" but "ruler," who can be either female or male or whatever. There is only one role that has a definite gender. That's the role of mom, which is always female.

What's the most beautiful part of a woman?

Some provincial parts of the world might say the face, or breasts, or legs. Ridiculous, say the Marquesans. It's a woman's vulva.

Thousands of miles from the closest continent, the Marquesas Islands are remote and spectacular. Black and white sand beaches, mountain cliffs along the sea, waterfalls taller than skyscrapers, sea-cave studded shores. It's a wild place where you can still be the first human into a deep valley, dense jungle, or volcanic mountain.

Okay, it's not all sweetness and light. Warring tribes used to enjoy dining on the enemy. A strict social hierarchy had a chief at the top. Yet Marquesans have always insisted everyone has inherent divinity and deserves respect. Add the great weather, yummy food—fish and crops grown in rich volcanic soil—and sea temps in the 80s year-round. There's a good reason Paul Gauguin (you know, the painter) hung out there.

Marquesans celebrate beauty and pleasure. They are famous for gorgeous, intricate tattoos that cover the entire bodies of both men and women.

As for pleasure—that's a no-brainer: sex! Men and women agree that both should desire and enjoy sex. The only taboo—your relatives.

Virginity and chastity? Don't be ridiculous. Sure, those rules are okay—for royalty—but normal folks should have a good time. Especially when they're young and unmarried. Older teens are known as "taure-are-a," between childhood and adulthood. *Taure-are-a* must have sexual adventures and lots of sexual liaisons. It's part of their nature. Besides, how else can you test potential mates? Later, they'll have to get married and become boring adults who have less fun.

Just don't wait too long. If a girl remains a virgin, blood will fill her head and body and drive her insane.

Best of all, practice makes perfect. And Marquesan men strive for perfection. The top priority is to make sure women enjoy the experience. Marquesan men pay special attention to vaginas. They say kissing a woman's lips is a bit gross. It's much more enjoyable and sanitary to kiss her "lower lips."

Young women also make the most of what heaven has bestowed. Girls learn to squeeze their vaginas during sex so they "wink, wink" *('amo 'amo)* to "make the loins rejoice."

Getting older is not a total zero. Sure, you only make love every other night instead of ten times per night like the normal nineteen-year-old. But age has its perks. Boys ask older, experienced women to help them remove the scab of ritual superincision, which can only be done by vigorous intercourse. (FYI, a superincision is kind of a partial circumcision, just a cut along the upper part of the penis foreskin from the tip to the corona.)

Only one behavior is considered sexually deviant: the celibate role of the priest, which conflicts with men's true nature.

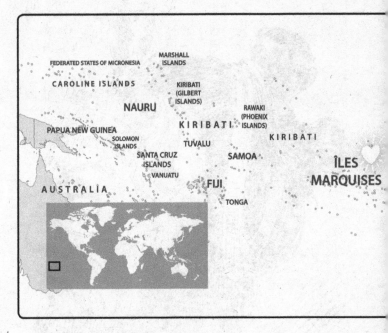

MARQUESAS ISLANDS

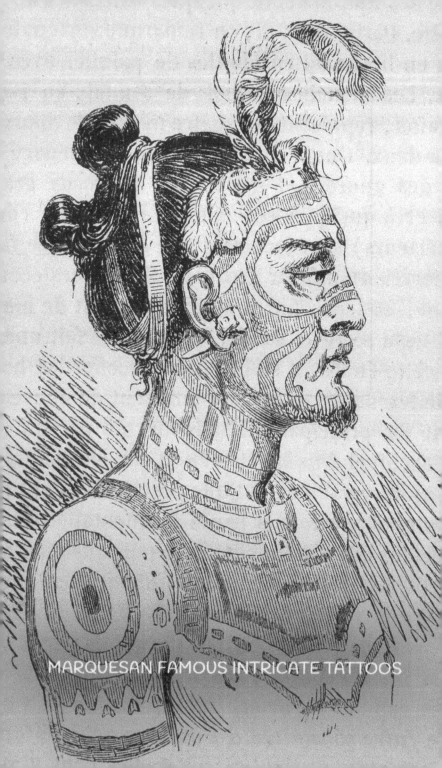

MARQUESAN FAMOUS INTRICATE TATTOOS

Wrestling for love

Mongol women are known for being strong, proud, and independent. No wonder. They come from a long line of super-dames, stretching back to the Mongol Empire of the thirteenth and fourteenth centuries. Those were rough times, as the Mongol armies swept across, pillaged, and conquered an area three times the size of the US.

Mongol women were in there swinging with the rest of the hordes. They were fierce warriors, powerful military commanders, mighty wrestlers, revered shaman, and clever businesspeople. Mongol men were hip to the women's sharp minds. A Mongol man always tried to marry an older woman so she could counsel him wisely. They knew any guy who didn't listen to his mom's or wife's advice was just defensive and immature.

At the height of Mongol power, women brilliantly ruled the empire. Take Queen Mandhuhai, who led the battles that brought the Mongols their greatest success. At one point, she decided she should pass on the family name. She married a cute, much younger prince and had eight kids, all while leading Mongol armies in battle.

Another Mongol lady badass was Princess Khutulun, great-great-granddaughter of Genghis Khan. Khutulun was famous as a kind of Freddy-Krueger-cum-super-soldier, who terrified the enemy, and a savvy battle strategist for King Kaidu, her dad. Coleridge really should have written poems about her instead of her uncle Kublai Khan.

Khutulun's parents applauded her chosen profession of soldier, but eventually suggested their superheroine marry. Khutulun thought that sounded lame. To jazz it up, she challenged suitors to a game with high stakes. The hubby-hopefuls had to wrestle her. He wins, she marries him. She wins, he hands over one hundred horses.

Loads of eager men. Loads of losers. She ended up with ten thousand horses and no hubby. Perfect!

But even badasses get the blues. Khutulun finally decided to marry. She picked a cute guy, told him to skip the wrestling bout, and they tied the knot.

When her father wanted to make her Khan, she said she didn't want the desk job. Instead, she handed Khan-ship to her brother and she became commander-in-chief of the army.

Today, Khutulun's impact on wrestling lives on. Over the centuries, guys scared of losing to a woman made wrestling men-only. They forced all contenders to fight in bare-chest wrestling shirts to prove they are guys, not hotshot women stealing into the ring to beat them up.

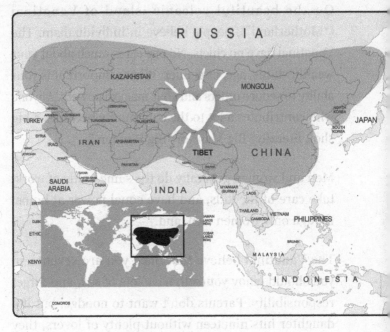

MONGOL EMPIRE

Happy meals for real

On the beautiful volcanic island of Vanatinai ("Motherland"), people believe in individualism. The Vanatinai have no chiefs. No one cares much about your wealth, status, age, or gender. What's important is your ability to seduce others and your magical powers. Anyone who contributes a lot to the community becomes a big shot, literally "Big Man" or "Big Woman."

Men and women generally do the same kinds of work, take care of the kids, and have equal power at home, though only women own land.

The Vanatinai believe that once you are seventeen, you should enjoy yourself, have lots of sex, and forget responsibility. Parents don't want to noodge, but if a daughter hits nineteen without plenty of lovers, they begin to worry, "Where did we go wrong?"

Before marriage, women figure it's best to have a variety of lovers. You must have sex with the same guy at least twice to get pregnant, so sleeping around is just sensible birth control. If, by chance, prevention fails, no worries. Your mom's clan will enthusiastically welcome your children as new members.

If a woman invites a guy to have an affair, he has to decide where they meet: in the woods or in her parents' home after everyone's in bed. Plus side of her bed: comfort. Plus side of the woods: way cheaper. If they sleep in her home, her mom will make him "fill a basket" with valuables after a night of naked fun. He wouldn't dare refuse, terrified she'll sic bad juju on him.

Ah well, affairs might be pricey, but the wedding ceremony is cheap. If she agrees to marry, he seals the deal simply by cooking breakfast. Share a meal, you're hitched.

Of course, post-wedding is a little tougher. The new groom must do "bride service." He works free for his mother-in-law for up to a year. Then, if he wins mom-in-law's approval, the couple can spend some time at his mom's home.

If married life isn't bliss, either spouse can initiate divorce as cheaply and simply as they married. The Vanatinai say both marriage and divorce should be easy, because you may have to do them often until you find "the one."

Does it work? You decide. Violence is extremely rare among the Vanatinai. Rape and sexual assault are completely unknown.

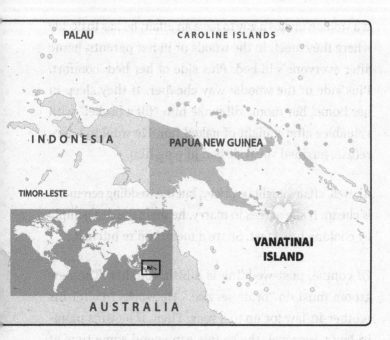

VANATINAI ISLAND OF PAPUA NEW GUINEA

Marriage
AND OTHER
MYSTERIES

Choosing your spouse is your basic right. We all agree: young people resent parents controlling their match.

Not so fast...

A bright, gorgeous young friend of mine in Rajasthan, India, was being married by her parents to a slow, goofy, rather odd-looking, mildly pleasant man. I expected some wistfulness, at least, from this great beauty, but was surprised to get only a lighthearted shrug. "He's kind," she smiled, "and works hard. I doubt I can pick better."

But that was a small town in Rajasthan. Surely, the urbane, worldly young people in Bombay and Delhi want to rebel against this violation of their basic human rights. In Bombay, I got my answer.

Ravi was smart, ambitious, handsome, articulate, sophisticated, and thoughtful. At twenty-five, he owned and ran a luxury jewelry store in a Bombay five-star hotel. At first, I stopped to admire the gorgeous baubles in the window. As we became friends, we'd sip tea and chat during lulls between customers. We talked about our lives, the differences—and similarities—between the US and India, our plans and hopes for the future. Finally I raised the delicate question—he would select his own bride, wouldn't he?

He smiled at this most American of questions. "Of course, my parents will choose a wife for me," he replied cheerily.

"Really?" I spluttered, shocked. "But...why? Don't you want to choose your own wife?"

His tone was serene and assured: "I'm young. What do I know about women? My mother understands women very well and she loves me. She is far better suited to pick a good wife for me than I could pick for myself." He grinned, "And if something goes wrong, I won't feel that I was the one who made the mistake."

Years later, as I suffered through a divorce, I wondered if he might be right. One thing was clear from my travels: there are oh-so-many ways to tie those lovely bonds of marriage.

Only gold diggers need apply

Marital problems? Call the Turu of Tanzania. They'll explain that love and marriage just don't compute. A loveless, but prosperous, marriage works best.

The Turu fun starts with boys' puberty festivals. Lovers of all ages join the main event: dancing as tight and sexy as possible. Everyone sings the old favorites, praising the penis, the vagina, and all types of sexual fun. The aim is to warm up the dancing partners—who'd better not be married—to have stoking-hot sex that night.

The Turu say it's fine to fall in love—just not with your spouse. Marriage, after all, is a business deal. Husband and wife stay together as long as they're prospering. They even encourage one another to take lovers (*mbuyu*). That's the best way to keep messy emotions where they should be—in love affairs—so they don't endanger the matrimonial bottom line.

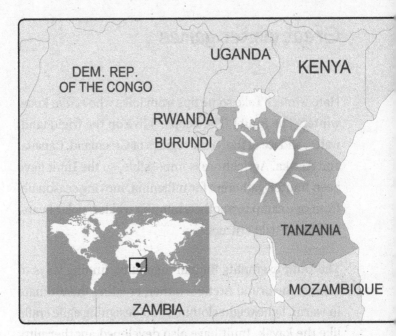

TURU OF TANZANIA

Great winter games

Hate winter? Take some tips from folks who *really* know winter. The Inuit ("The People") live on the frigid land, water, and ice of the Arctic regions of Greenland, Canada, and Alaska. Agriculture is impossible, so the Inuit have been hunter-gatherers for millennia, moving seasonally from one camp to another, hunting whales, polar bears, and other wild critters.

The Inuit exemplify human ingenuity, finding ways to survive the brutal Arctic weather, creating the ultimate in warm, lightweight clothing, and designing agile crafts like the kayak. Inuit have also developed another nifty solution for those long, cold, dark Arctic winters: be neighborly!

One great way to build that neighborhood spirit is "wife swapping"—or better call it "husband swapping" since only the guys had to move to another house. Of course, not all Inuit communities do things the same way.

There are uptight ones in North Alaska, who have lots of rules: No swapping with close relatives. No swapping just for fun. No swapping in secret. Swap only to expand your network of distant relatives, because all of the kids born after the swap are "half-brothers" and "half-sisters," even if they have no biological connection. Aim to swap with folks in potentially dangerous neighborhoods. That way, you have relatives who can help if you get stuck in a tough hood.

Other Inuit groups, say in Greenland, have had a different take. Picture this. It's another cold, dark night in a long winter. Times are tough. Game is scarce. Lamp oil is limited. Morale is low.

Why whine about it? Might as well make the best of the situation. Raise morale and economize on lamp oil with a traditional "extinguishing-the-lamp" game. Sort of a combo musical chairs, prayer meeting, and Roman orgy.

Invite several other couples over to your igloo. Have the *angakkuq* (shaman) communicate with the spirits to create the right mood. Everyone get naked. Put out the lamps. In the complete darkness, fumble around until everyone has a partner. Do what comes naturally. Eventually, stumble back to your spouse. Re-light the lamps. Enjoy the resulting warm, relaxed and jovial atmosphere.

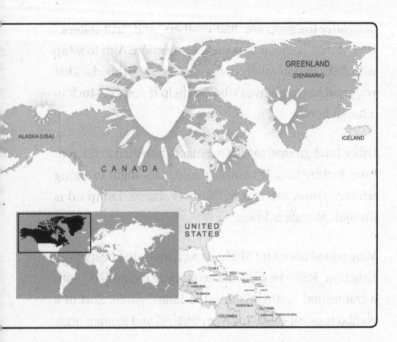

INUIT OF GREENLAND, CANADA AND ALASKA

I'll always be true to you, darling, in my fashion...

In villages along their Melanesian sugar-white beaches and crystalline blue seas, Lesu husbands and wives divvy up the chores—farming, fishing, cooking, caring for the kids, taking lots of lovers. Sleep with only your spouse? That is *too weird*, say the Lesu, especially when you're young. Nothing's more suspicious than a faithful wife. "What's wrong with her?" hubby wonders. "*Normal* wives have plenty of lovers."

Want your Lesu neighbors to think you're *really a* pervert? Stay faithful to your spouse for years.

In the valleys of Sikkim's towering Kanchenjunga mountain range, the Róng agree. Normal spouses sleep around. These peaceful, shy, deeply religious people live close to nature, farming and tending livestock. The Róng believe aggression and conflict are bizarre. Normal people want to make love, not war. Snow-bound winter or wildflower spring—anytime's the right time to take a lover.

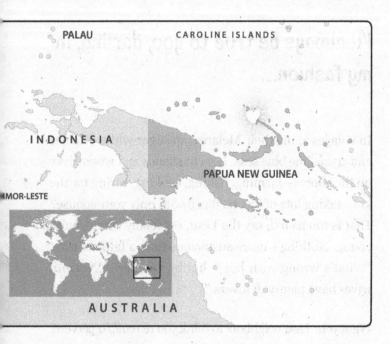

LESU OF PAPUA NEW GUINEA

The Róng take "Be your brother's keeper" to heart. Wives have full freedom to sleep with their husbands' younger brothers. Ditto for husbands and their wives' younger sisters.

The Róng language has no word for jealousy. Sex, they say, is like food and drink. Of course you love a home-cooked meal. But it's always fun to dine out once in awhile.

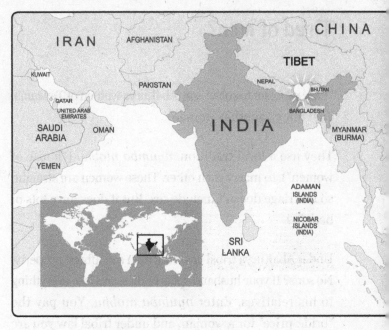

RÓNG OF SIKKIM, INDIA

Tired of men?

"Easy problem to solve!" say AbaKurya women of Tanzania. Just marry another woman.

They use a local tradition, *nyumba ntobhu* ("house of women"), to marry each other. These women are straight, so marriage doesn't include sex. But it does have lots of benefits.

Under AbaKurya tribal law, only men can inherit property. No sons? If your husband splits or dies, you lose everything to his relatives. Enter *nyumba ntobhu*. You pay the "bride-price" for a woman, and under tribal law you are married. Your "wife" takes lovers, aiming to have a son for your marriage. Succeed and you keep your property, which you can leave to him.

Nyumba ntobhu has other charms. It gives women— especially widows, women without children, and divorced women—a loving, stable family. No wonder female couples make up 10 to 15 percent of AbaKurya households.

Plenty of men also like the arrangement. Sex with no obligations: win-win.

Of course, nothing's simple. Tanzanian law doesn't recognize the AbaKurya *nyumba ntobhu*. But men rarely try to fight tribal law. No one wants to tangle with tribal elders. It's easier just to find a woman who wants to marry *you*, not your sister.

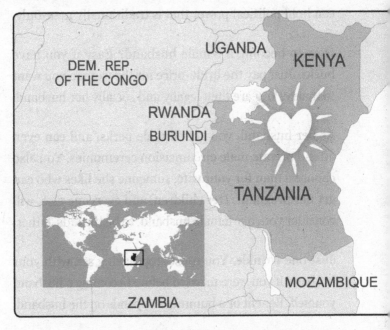

ABAKURYA OF TANZANIA AND KENYA

The Nandi, of eastern Kenya, agree with the AbaKurya. Behind every successful woman is...another woman.

Like the AbaKurya, the Nandi union is nonsexual. But women are not just protecting their property. They become "husbands" to get the political power and privileges of men.

Like women in the USA, Nandi women have a tough time winning political office no matter how smart and skilled they are. The solution: become a "man." That way, she can hold political power that is traditionally men-only.

How to become a female husband? Easy if you have bucks. Just pay the bride-price for the woman you want to marry. You are then legally and socially her husband.

As her husband, you get all male perks, and can even attend private male circumcision ceremonies. You also choose a man for your wife, someone she likes who can get her pregnant. Her children, and everyone else, will consider you, her female husband, to be the kids' father.

Just one wrinkle. You must stop having sex with your husband if you were married before becoming a husband yourself. Benefit or a bummer—depends on the husband.

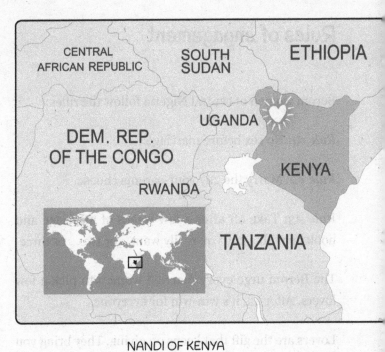

NANDI OF KENYA

Rules of engagement

Berom women of central Nigeria follow the rules:

Rule #1: No sex before marriage.

Rule #2: Marry the guy your parents choose.

Rule #3: Take off after a few weeks of marriage and hook up with a guy you really want... or two... or three.

The Berom urge every married woman to pick a few lovers. After all, it's win-win for everyone.

Lovers are the gift that keeps on giving. They bring you money and presents year after year. They even help you with the farming and other chores. What could be better? It's social security plus lots of fun sex.

No need to sneak around. Your lover's wife? No problem! You'll be friends, practically sisters. She'll help you if times get tough. You're always there for her. The kids should also be good friends, and work and play together.

Your lovers will woo your husband, too. Gifts, money, loans, or whatever will please him, every year. Hubby figures, "We might as well be buddies." After all, they have a mutual interest—you.

Besides, he gets to be the lover of other men's wives. Plus, an ambitious man needs followers. And the best followers are—you guessed it—his wife's lovers and his mistresses' husbands.

Best of all, he avoids a divorce. Better to give you plenty of space for new friends, lovers and romantic adventures than have you dump him.

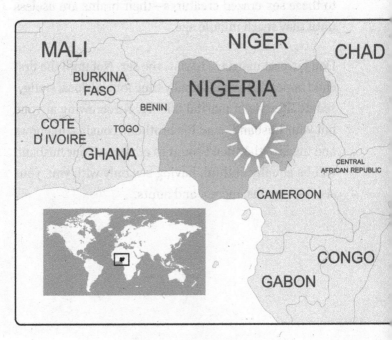

BEROM OF NIGERIA

127

All in the family...

The Chuukese of the Chuuk Islands live in a paradise of endless white sand beaches framing warm, translucent, green waters. The Chuukese are practical people who follow the rules of Mother Nature. One clear rule is that teenagers think only of sex. Teen virginity? Not only worthless, but impossible for kids over seventeen. Might as well tell them to fly. No use trying to teach anything to these sex-crazed creatures—their brains are useless until they reach middle age.

Don't expect marriage to slow the sex. Not until the first child appears. Then it's finally time for a serious, stodgy, sedate lifestyle of marital fidelity. No screwing anyone but your husband...and his brothers, cousins, nephews and uncles—they don't count as adultery. Your husband will be equally faithful, having sex only with you, your sisters, cousins, nieces, and aunts.

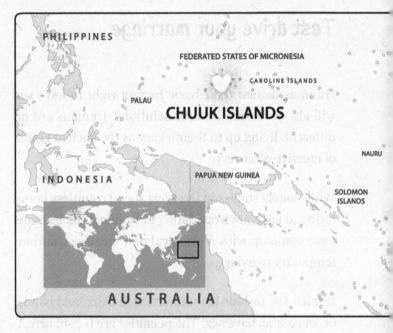

THE CHUUKESE, CHUUK ISLANDS

Test drive your marriage

Humans denied their basic human right to have sex will always devise creative solutions. Iranians are no different, living up to their legacy as the ancient cradle of creative discovery.

While lonely singles in the West spend countless hours trying to navigate from dating to bedding, the Iranians have come up with a practical and creative solution: temporary marriage.

Iranian law forbids the unmarried to date, hold hands, or, of course, have sex. The penalties are harsh: arrest, fines, even flogging. But as with so many government rules, there is a loophole.

Under Shiite Islamic law, you can contract for a temporary marriage (*sigheh*). The terms are straightforward, sort of like renting an apartment: the length of the union, the bridewealth amount the groom will pay the bride, proof you're both single. You can try out the marriage for a few hours, months, or years. When the contract ends, the woman must wait two menstrual cycles before she remarries. Oh, and she must be Muslim (preferably Shiite because Sunni Islam outlaws temp marriage). If things go well, you may decide to proceed to permanent matrimony. Meanwhile, if the morality police stop you, you can show your official marriage certificate.

Iran is just as tech-crazy as everywhere else. You can find your temp spouse on the Web. Just sort by looks, wealth, health, financial stability, "veil status" for women (how much face does she show in public), and car price for men (cars are a major status symbol in Iran). Think this is a fringe movement? Think again. The major website, Hafezoon, boasts more than 100,000 users.

The only downside is the site's ban on same-sex connections. Once you set your gender in a profile, you can only search for those of the "opposite" sex.

Think this is all some new craze? Wrong. The roots of Shiite temporary marriage go way back. Some Islamic scholars trace its origins to the seventh century, the beginning of the Islamic Golden Age, while Europe was still in the Dark Ages.

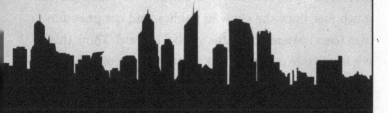

شبکه اجتماعی حافظون

وَ لَقَدْ خَلَقْنَا الْإِنْسَانَ وَ نَعْلَمُ مَا تُوَسْوِسُ بِهِ نَفْسُهُ وَ نَحْنُ أَقْرَبُ إِلَيْهِ مِنْ حَبْلِ الْوَرِيدِ (ق.١٦)
ما انسان را آفریدیم و وسوسه های نفس او را می دانیم، و ما به او از رگ قلبش نزدیکتریم!

همسریابی ازدواج موقت و صیغه یابی در سایت حافظون

حافظون، یک پایگاه اختصاصی برای همسریابی برای ازدواج موقت است. هدف این سایت، تشکیل یک جامعه مجازی برای خانها و آقایان مجردیست که موفق به ازدواج دائم نشده و قصد
ازدواج موقت دارند. لازم بذکر است که حافظون یک موسسه همسریابی نمی باشد و لذا فردی را به فرد دیگر معرفی نمیکند. همچنین حافظون وابسته به هیچ سازمان و نهادی نمی
به صورت مستقل اداره میشود.

HAFEZOON TEMPORARY MARRIAGE WEBSITE

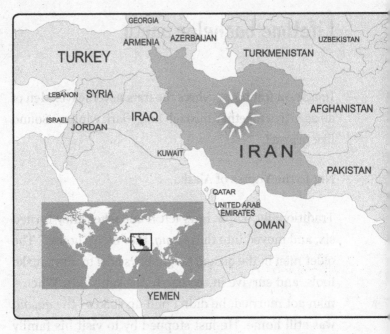

IRAN

Lifetime bachelor party

Imagine a frat house where the frats never leave. Men of all ages live together through long, dark winters. Sound like prison?

Not to the Yupiks of Alaska.

Traditionally, Yupik boys left home when they turned six, and moved into the *qasqig*, the "men's house." The older men in the *qasqig* taught boys how to hunt, make tools, and survive in the harsh Alaskan wilds. When a man got married, he didn't pull up stakes—the *qasqig* was still home. He just stopped by to visit his family now and then...long enough to play with the kids and mess around with the wife. Of course, his wife and her girlfriends were always welcome to party at the men's festivals, ceremonies, and dances.

The women built their own house, the *ena*, near the *qasqig*. There, girls learned all the skills they'd need. Most crucial: to sew—because any man is doomed without a woman to sew for him. Clothes not only keep you warm on those -80°F days; they are the only way to keep evil spirits at bay. One tiny rip and demons can sneak in to nab you.

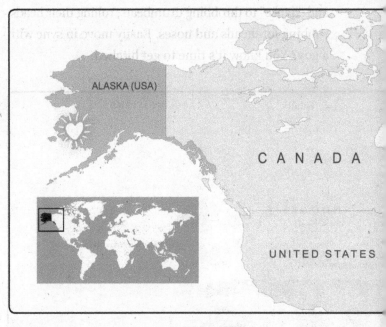

YUPIK OF ALASKA, USA

The Medlpa of New Guinea agree it's best for women and men to live separately. Young Medlpa boys move from mom's to the men's house, which is home for the rest of their lives. Women and girls live in the women's house, which is also home to the village pigs.

Still, the Medlpa believe in true love. An amorous man paints himself with pig fat dye and loads on jewelry of feathers and shells. He woos his beloved by composing and singing songs full of sexual innuendo. If she's impressed, they meet with several other couples to sit

Sex Rules!

and "dance" to throbbing drumbeats, rolling their heads, rubbing foreheads and noses. Easily move in sync with a guy? You know it's time to get hitched.

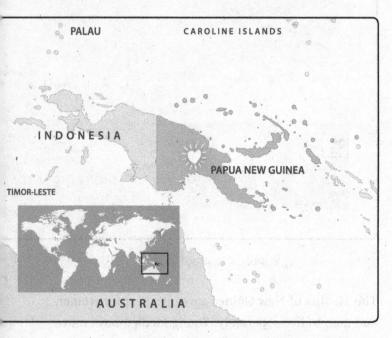

MEDLPA OF PAPUA NEW GUINEA

WEIRD USA MARRIAGE LAWS

At some point in their lives, most folks in the USA have lived with someone without being married. If that includes you, you're a criminal in some states. Florida, Michigan, Mississippi, and Virginia outlaw living with your main squeeze if you're not married.

But don't think getting married will let you off the hook.

Detroit, Michigan made it illegal for a man to frown at his wife on Sunday. Of course, it should have been everyday, but, hey, the legislators were men.

And for you, ladies… marry the same guy over and over in Kentucky and you've got more than psychological problems. Kentucky makes it illegal to marry the same man more than three times.

Once you're hitched, better stick to the straight and narrow. If you engage in adultery, you're an outlaw in eighteen states, some with pretty hefty penalties:

Oklahoma – up to five years in prison and up to $500 fine.

Massachusetts - up to three years in prison or a $500 fine. If you were married but now are divorced and still living together, sorry. You're still guilty and can end up in the slammer.

Wisconsin – up to three years in jail and up to $10,000 fine.

Idaho – up to three years behind bars and up to $1,000 fine.

Minnesota – up to one year in jail and up to $3,000 fine.

Illinois – up to one year in jail for the cheating spouse. The lover gets a year, too.

Georgia – up to one year in jail or up to $1,000 fine.

Mississippi – up to six months in jail and up to $500 fine.

Utah – up to six months in jail and up to $1,000 fine.

South Carolina – six months to a year behind bars and $500 - $1,000 fine.

New York – up to three months in jail.

Florida – up to two months in jail and up to $500 fine.

Arizona – one month in jail for both the cheating spouse and the lover.

Kansas – one month in jail and up to $500 fine.

North Carolina – up to one month in jail.

Virginia – up to $250 fine.

Michigan – maybe jail or something…

Maryland – the same penalty whether you go to a movie or totally get it on with someone who's not your spouse. Ten buck fine.

The first "Wives Club"

In the ancient forests, towering mountains, and spectacular sea cliffs of South Africa's Wild Coast, the people are friendly. Pondo women, especially, love to be helpful. They are always ready to lend each other a hand: watch the kids, help weed the garden, arrange an extramarital affair....

Want to spice up your love life? This is the place to be. The Pondo women—even your sisters-in-law—will pitch right in. They'll scout out sexy lovers. Arrange a rendezvous. Keep your husband busy while you're off to a clandestine tryst. If hubby whines—ignore him! The women figure their affairs are perfectly proper. No sense letting a jealous husband spoil good, clean fun.

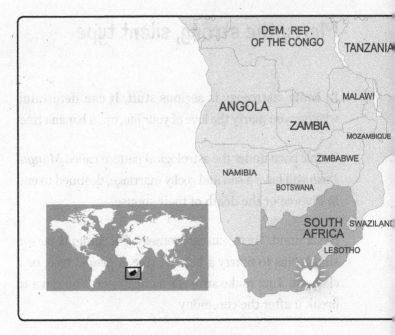

PONDO OF SOUTH AFRICA

Marry the strong, silent type

In India, astrology is serious stuff. It can determine whether you marry the love of your life, or...a banana tree!

People born under the astrological pattern called *Mangal Dosh* will have a sad and rocky marriage, destined to end in divorce or the death of their spouse.

Never mind. There's an easy remedy. The *Manglik* person simply has to marry a banana tree, a peepal tree, or a clay pot. Just make sure it's a cheap pot. You have to break it after the ceremony.

Want to be super safe? Follow the lead of famous Indian actress Aishwarya Rai. She married not one, but two trees because she is *Manglik*. The trees didn't seem to mind, but lawyers later sued her for "entering a false marriage."

Eventually—perhaps after divorcing said trees—she was safe to marry her fiancé, heartthrob actor Abhishek Bachchan.

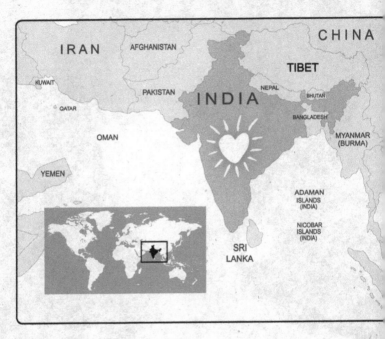

INDIA

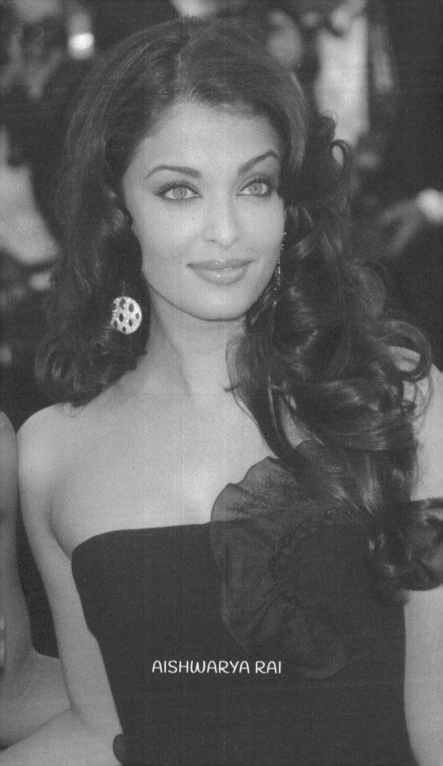

AISHWARYA RAI

Love, better than a blanket...

The Innu have lived in the rugged, pristine subarctic forest of *Nitassinan* (northeast Quebec and eastern Labrador) for thousands of years. Until the 1700s, the Innu practiced polygamy, and both wives and husbands had complete sexual freedom after marriage.

The women thought this worked just fine. After all, they outnumbered the men. The new-fangled idea the missionaries brought—just one wife per man—was absurd. If a man could only marry one woman, some women would be left out in the cold. What woman would ever agree to such a stupid idea?

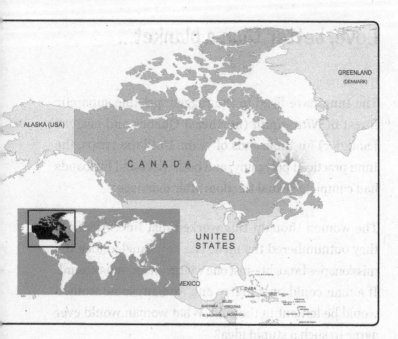

INNU OF CANADA

Meetin' in the Garden of Eatin'

The Nagovisi of South Bougainville, Papua New Guinea, live in a world of magnificent rainforests, active volcanoes, spectacular coral reefs, and freedom. Especially the freedom to have sex with—and marry—anyone you like... and as often as you like.

If you both enjoyed the rolls in the woods, it's time for a "trial marriage"—easy to do, and easy to end if the glow goes. Or maybe get "a little bit" married. A couple has a nice church wedding, lives together, has a child—but of course they're not *really* married. Not until he works in her garden.

Only women can own land, so *real* marriage begins when she lets you help her with the farming. You start weeding, you're really hitched. Only then can you eat from the garden.

So, guys, remember your motto: a happy wife, a happy life, and a happy belly.

A contented wife lets you help farm and eat the crops. Got a job? She may even let you keep a little of your salary.

An unhappy wife won't kick you out of the bedroom. Way worse. She'll ban you from the garden...and eating the crops. Then you have three choices. Make up, go back to Mom's, or starve.

Still, divorce is rare after kids are born. And it's never about adultery. After all, everyone knows it's impossible for any woman and man to spend time alone without having sex. Plus, married couples can't screw during pregnancy and for two years after the birth. So you can get it on like bunnies every couple of years, but what about in-between?

What do you *think*?

Luckily, you can never get pregnant from an affair. After all, it takes repeated sex with the same person to get pregnant, and adulterous affairs are but brief. So no worries on that score.

But getting caught *is* embarrassing and you might even have to pay a fine. So stick to a time-honored solution: find a lover for your spouse. That way, if you get caught, you can call it even. And, if you're a guy, even keep eating.

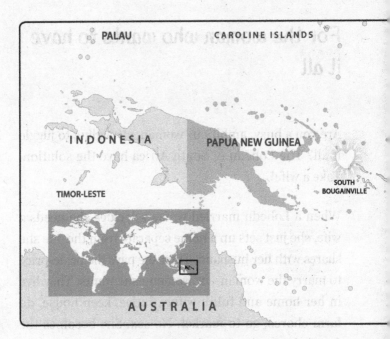

NAGOVISI OF SOUTH BOUGAINVILLE,
PAPUA NEW GUINEA

For the woman who wants to have it all

Are you a busy, ambitious woman, struggling to juggle it all? The Lobedu of South Africa have the solution. Take a wife!

When a Lobedu married woman decides she needs a wife, she just sets up a home separate from the one she shares with her husband. Then she pays the bride-price to marry the woman—or women—she wants. They live in her home and fulfill wifely duties, keep house, do farm chores, go to market. No sex. She becomes the female-husband of *her* home, and remains the wife of *her husband's* home.

Not surprising that the Lobedu hatched this optimal solution. There, women dominate politics. They have had powerful ruling queens for hundreds of years. Their Rain Queen can control rainfall—nice talent in parched lands. She also has several wives. One famous queen had nine. No worries that other local rulers might mess with her. Everybody needs rain.

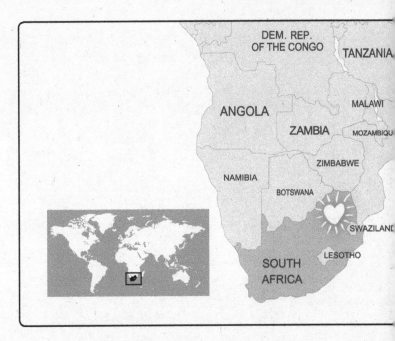

LOBEDU OF SOUTH AFRICA

Foxy
LAD(Y) OR DRESS
FOR SUCCESS

Everywhere, "men's" and "women's" dress codes are strictly enforced. There are clothes forbidden to men. Ditto for women. Breaking the code can inflame society's fury. Yet the codes vary wildly from place to place and often contradict each other.

In India, I immediately knew the clothes for me—a long cloth called a *lungi* (*lung-ee*) to wrap around my waist, making a long, loose skirt that protected my legs from the blistering sun while letting in the passing breezes. A loose, long-sleeved, cotton blouse called a "*kurta*," with the same advantages. They were protective, cool and comfy, perfect for India's intense heat. They were also "men's clothes."

It took a little longer for my mate to switch from his t-shirt and jeans to the same "skirt and blouse." When we returned home, he continued to wear them during Boston's sweltering summers...but never in public.

Sometimes things got looser. On an isolated beach in south India, where I spent one lovely winter, I usually wore nothing at all. Living on the beach and swimming the warm, crystalline, tranquil Arabian Sea, required neither bathing suit nor clothes. If anyone appeared or I had to go to the village, a half-hour walk away, I simply tied a *lungi* around my neck.

In towns where my "men's clothes" of skirt and blouse (*lungi* and *kurta)* scandalized, I switched to a *salwar-kameez*, a loose, knee-length tunic over pantaloons. The *salwar kameez* is a testimony to the genius of Indian women—super-comfortable, cool, easy to fit, looks great. In India, it's formal enough for a business meeting or dinner party. Women of the West unite! You have nothing to lose but those miserable suits and heels!

Don't be a yahoo, be a Mahu!

Boys learn early not to be "girly." A guy in women's clothes—skirt, stockings, high heels, makeup—will draw laughs...or worse.

But not in Polynesia.

For centuries, villagers in the tropical paradise of Polynesian islands delighted in their transvestites—called *mahus* in Tahiti and Hawai'i, *fa'afafine* in Samoa, *fakaleiti* in Tonga. Take Tahiti's *mahus*. They plucked out the hair on their faces and dressed, danced, and sang like women. They could weave and paint cloth, make mats, and do other "women's" work.

Tahitian villagers bragged about their *mahus*. It's wonderful, they said, to see someone who blends the essence of male and female, unites *yin* and *yang*. Finally! A man who can do women's work!

Like other Polynesians, Tahitians prized transvestites as good luck charms, and every village wanted one of their very own. Only a village of losers lacked its own transvestite.

Even royalty hoped some of that good fortune would smile on them. Hawai'i's King Kamehameha pleaded with transvestites to live near his home, to bring him luck.

Today, wherever Polynesian tradition holds firm, they continue to honor their *mahus*. So...want your hometown to be prosperous, desirable, and classy? Get yourselves a *mahu*.

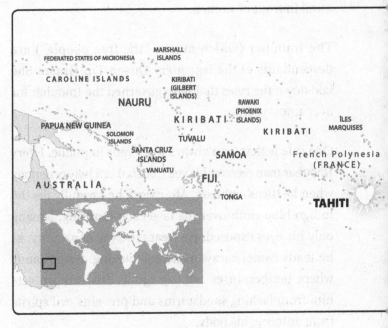

TAHITI

Hate that suit and tie?

Lighten up! You could be an Imouhar!

These men of the central Sahara never leave home without it—their veils, that is. These fierce and courageous fighters, who live by a strict code of honor, always wear a veil in front of women.

The Imouhar (which means "the free people") are descendants of the legendary Queen Tin Hinan. She laid down the rules that have governed the Imouhar for over 1,500 years.

One rule is that men always wear veils in public. Every Imouhar man receives his veil (*Alasho*) in a holy ceremony when he turns eighteen. Afterward, he carefully fits the indigo blue cloth over his face each morning, leaving only his eyes exposed. He wears the veil constantly, as he leads camel caravans across blazing desert sands where temperatures can top 130°F. His veil protects him from lashing sandstorms and prevents evil spirits from entering his body.

He even wears it inside his leather tent—sometimes even when he sleeps. At meals, he lifts the veil just high enough to slip the food between his lips. No self-respecting Imouhar man would let a woman—worst of all, a lover—ever get the tiniest glimpse of his mouth.

Imouhar women don't bother wearing veils at all. Be sensible, say the Imouhar, everyone benefits from seeing women's beautiful faces.

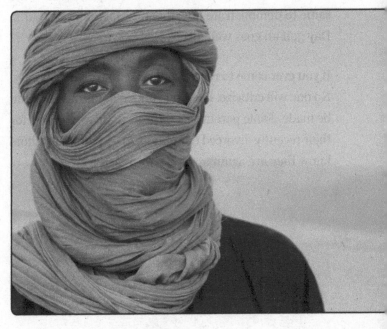

IMOUHAR MAN

Young people find and choose their own marriage partners, though their parents must give the final okay. Women have equal rights within the union. They also own most of the property—the tents, all possessions inside, and all the animals except the camels. The men get the camels.

After the wedding, the bride and groom must spend three days and nights without leaving their tent. No wild sexual romp here. On Day 1, she declines him. As a good husband, he respects her wishes completely and dedicates himself to making her comfortable. Day 2, more of the same to demonstrate how much he loves her so that…. Day 3, if all goes well, fireworks!

If you ever come to regret your selection, divorce is easy. No one will criticize. Everyone understands mistakes can be made. Some parents even throw a "divorce party" for their recently divorced daughters, to let potential suitors know they are again available for marriage.

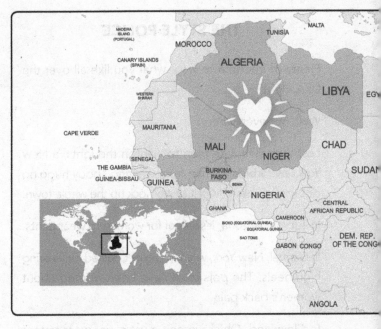

IMOUHAR OF ALGERIA, BURKINA FASO, LIBYA, MALI AND NIGER

THE STYLE POLICE

Plenty of freedom to wear what you like all over the USA, right?

Well, not everywhere…

Lest they stimulate men to wanton thoughts, a New York law forbids women from wearing "body hugging clothing" publicly. Might as well lock up the whole town.

In Tucson, Arizona, it's illegal for women to wear pants.

In Carmel, New York, women can get busted for wearing high heels. The pols must have been worried about women's back pain.

In Cleveland, Ohio, women must never wear patent leather shoes in public. No doubt wanting to maintain the city's high standards for style.

Not to worry, guys, they haven't forgotten you. In Miami, Florida, men can get busted for wearing a strapless gown in public. So stick to gowns with straps.

Life is better in free-swinging Walnut, CA. There, a man is free to dress as a woman – as long as he gets the sheriff's permission first.

Then there's the possibility of shucking the clothes altogether. Not in some places. Florida has a law against showering nude.

Oregon seconds that idea. To bathe legally, you must wear clothes that cover you, neck to knees.

Who wears the nose rings in your family?

If you're from Alaska, it's probably Grandpa. The men of some Inuit tribes wore elaborate jewelry, especially lip ornaments, right up to the twentieth century. Men had holes cut into the corners of their mouths, then stretched them to hold large pieces of ivory, stones, even coal or glass stoppers. One hot look was a small walrus tusk sticking out of each side of the mouth.

Guys, parents giving you a hard time about piercing? Remind them that pierced ears bring a long life and a ticket into heaven, according to the desert tribes of the North American Great Basin.

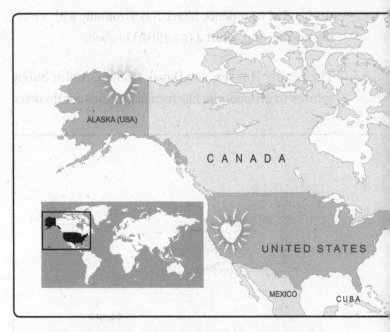

INUIT OF ALASKA AND NORTH AMERICAN DESERT
TRIBES OF NORTH AMERICA GREAT BASIN

Crave something more exotic? Try nipple-piercing like
Caesar's Roman centurions, who wore nipple rings to
show that they were macho, fearless, and fertile.

Not edgy enough?

Check out Apadravya or Palang piercing, popular with
the men of the Iban, Kayan, Kenyah, Kelabit, Dayak, and
other Sarawak tribes in Borneo. Not much to it. Just take

the head of your penis, pierce it horizontally with a nice, big needle, and insert a (smallish) barbell.

The result? Hot sex, say Dayak women. And if hubby refuses to get one, she has formal grounds for divorce.

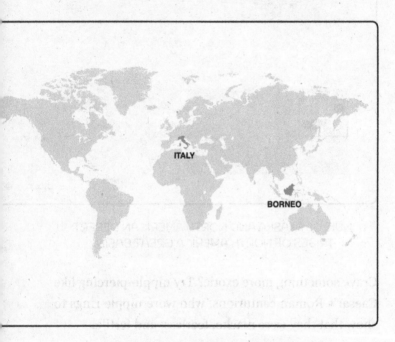

ROMAN CENTURIANS OF ROME, ITALY
AND DAYAK TRIBES OF BORNEO

Classic styles for men

Closet tired? Fill it with classics: decorative penis sheaths. They're all the rage in parts of Africa, South America, and the South Pacific Islands. Take a tip from the Bafia of Cameroon. A fashionable Bafia man has a penis sheath for every occasion: palm leaves for everyday. Snake or lizard skin with claws for steppin' out at night.

The well-dressed Amahuaca of Peru, the Brazilian Tupari, and the Ngqika of South Africa never go anywhere without their penis sheaths. The Tupari are serious. A good Tupari *never* removes his sheath in front of others—even for bathing. The Tupari considers Europeans, who bathe in the nude, quite disgusting—might as well be a monkey. In South Africa, a Ngqika who removes his or someone else's penis sheath will be fined.

Afraid it might clash with the rest of your wardrobe? Not to worry—you have lots to choose from. Best take a tip from the Dani of Papua New Guinea and have a wardrobe full of penis sheaths. Say, a long straight sheath for Saturday night, or a curved gourd sheath for special occasions. Of course, like any high fashion, it takes a little effort to put on. You simply whip out your handy boar tusk and shoehorn that baby into the sheath. Then stow the tusk in your hair for ready access in case your buddy slips out of its case.

Okay, your sheath might chafe a bit, but stop whining. Women have been suffering to stay fashionable for centuries.

There is always the comfy option: a nice Turkana loin skirt from Kenya that hangs in front of your boys and has a cozy pouch for the penis.

Or take a tip from the Japanese. Shinto priests discovered penis packaging in the eighth century and raised it to an art. Just slip the little dude into a *Kokigami*, a paper package shaped as some animal that turns you on. Then you and your partner can play out the sexual fantasies the animal inspires.

Going off to war? No problem. The amaXhosa of South Africa have a nice war-gourd with chains...and for that special guy, small bells can be attached.

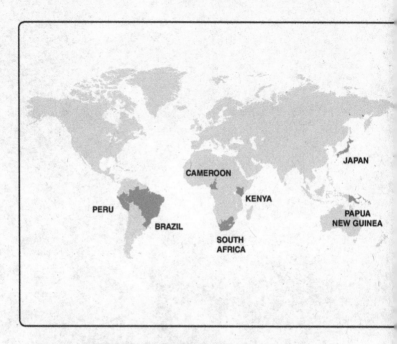

TRIBES USING PENIS SHEATHS
BAFIA IN CAMEROON, AMAHUACA IN PERU, TUPARI IN
BRAZIL, NGQIKA AND AMAXHOSA IN SOUTH AFRICA,
TURKANA IN KENYA, JAPANESE, DANI AND OTHERS IN
PAPUA NEW GUINEA

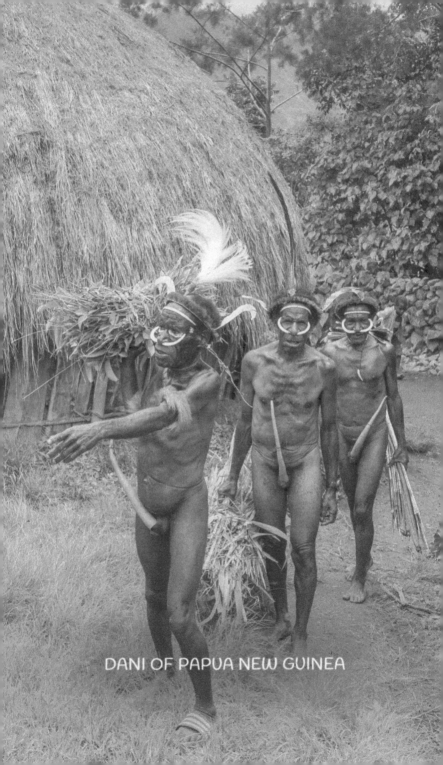

DANI OF PAPUA NEW GUINEA

The World's best-dressed choirboys...

In Tamil Nadu, at the southern tip of India, only the most talented Kaniyan singers and dancers get to perform in the celebration of the God Sudalai, protector of the dispossessed. And only men qualify for these top jobs. The lucky chosen dancers always wear their "Sunday best." First, they decorate their long, flowing hair in flowers. Then they add plenty of makeup, perfumed powder, and jewelry. For the final touch, they make "breasts" of balled up paper to wear beneath their blouses.

In their best falsetto voices, the singers praise God Sudalai and beg the spirit to enter a male dancer who can talk directly to the gods (*"komarathadigal"*). He spins wildly for hours, possessed by the divine spirit.

Singing and dancing all day for a god is tough work—no time left for a paying job. Besides, as everyone knows, it's women's place to make the bucks.

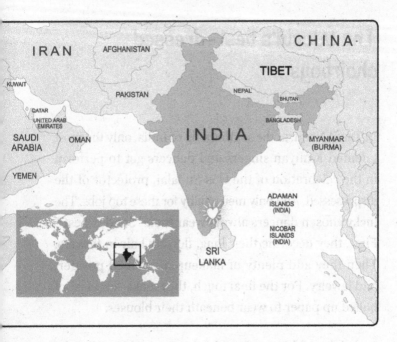

KANIYAN OF TAMIL NADU, INDIA

Redheads have more fun...

The tall, lean, handsome Moinjaang men of South Sudan know how to look hot, whether they're herding cattle along the White Nile river rapids or tending their grain fields. First, they dye their hair bright red using cattle piss. Then they shave their heads so there's just a tiny tuft of hair at the top. Using a thorn from an Acacia tree, they tease out every single curl of that little tuft.

Moinjaang women are just as chic. The fashionable Moinjaang woman shaves her eyebrows as well as her head. She leaves just a tiny hank of hair perched at the very top of her skull for the perfect "do."

The Moinjaang, also called Dinka, were once southern Sudan's richest and proudest tribe—many served as court judges and doctors. That is, until the 1990s when the government in Khartoum, North Sudan, and the Janjawid militia, brutally attacked the South, shattering lives and driving three million people to flee as refugees. Beauty, pride, and industriousness are no match for machine guns.

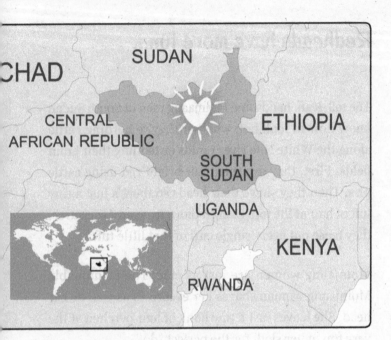

MOINJAANG OF SOUTH SUDAN

IN THE eye
OF THE BEHOLDER

"Beauty is in the eye of the beholder"—nothing's truer. I've seen blond hair trigger traffic accidents among thrilled men in India...and horrify village children in Melanesia. My blue eyes charm in some places and terrify in others. Old women in tiny rural villages have tried, out of pity, to rub off the white from my skin.

Some faraway beauty conventions echo the prejudices of home. In South India, a village headman's son pouted that his village had no pretty women. When I asked about one young beauty, he was mystified. Who could it be? When I pointed her out, he cringed. "Ridiculous," he spat, in a tone reserved for fools, "She is dark."

Mostly, though, notions of "beauty" are wildly different around the world. Women proudly flaunt earlobes that sag to their shoulders, lips that jut out like small plates, thoroughly shaven heads. Men parade deeply scarred faces, nostrils stretched to the size of baseballs, huge holes gouged into cheeks. These are the sirens and studs of their societies. The small, even features the West so adores are considered ugly to the point of deformity in many parts of the world.

My personal favorite are the Maasai. It seems a supremely decent and good-natured society to have standards of beauty anyone can attain simply by washing fairly often, cleaning teeth regularly with a twig, and standing with good posture.

During a safari led by Mingati, a Maasai friend from Nairobi, we stopped for a day in his village, a dusty collection of small, dark, circular huts made of mud, cow dung, branches, and straw. Flies wandered undisturbed across the faces and bodies of infants and toddlers sitting quietly alongside women grinding maize by hand, seemingly oblivious to the brutal heat. Their richly elaborate, lavishly woven jewelry was astonishing, like gemstones gleaming on a desert landscape.

Mingati had often told me of his wife's great beauty, and proudly introduced us. His wife, a slender young woman whose shaven head gleamed, wore a traditional blue Maasai cloth tied at the throat. Her neck was completely enveloped by intricately woven, brilliantly colored beaded necklaces. Long metal and beaded loops swung heavily from gaping holes at the top of her ears. Her ear lobes were tiny flesh threads around enormous holes hung with massive, beaded earrings. Her teeth were very white, with a large space in front where a tooth had been pulled to enhance her beauty.

When it comes to standards of "beauty," nothing is predictable.

Thankfully.

Somewhere in this world you're a perfect 10...

Whatever your looks, you are a fabulous beauty... You just need to be in the right place.

Cross-eyed? You're fairest in the land, say the Mayans of Mexico and Central America.

Thick, fat calves? Adorable, according to the Tiv of Nigeria.

No eyebrows or eyelashes? You're a true beauty, declare the Mongo of the Democratic Republic of Congo.

Sport just one single long eyebrow? You are the most gorgeous of women, argue the Syrians.

Rotund body with big buttocks and large, round legs? The Baganda of Uganda will lust after you.

Black teeth? The biggest turn-on, say the Yapese of Micronesia and the Lu of Vietnam.

Huge, protruding rear end? Makes you stunning, say the Khoikhoi of southern Africa—the bigger your butt, the more alluring.

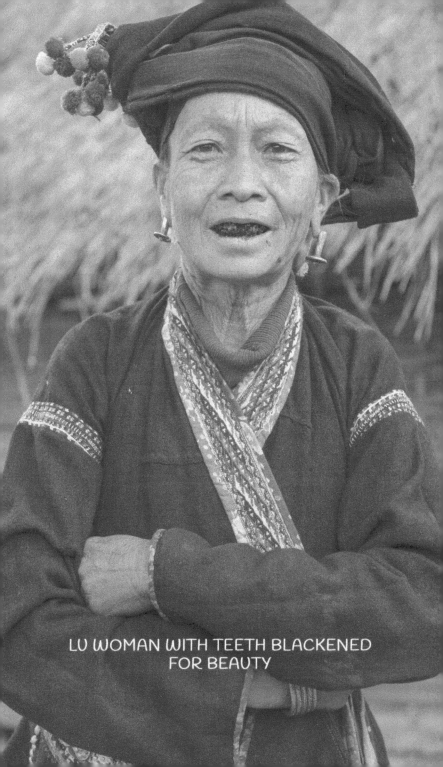

LU WOMAN WITH TEETH BLACKENED
FOR BEAUTY

Head a bit flattened? You will charm any man, insist the Kwakiutl of Canada.

Bulbous stomach and big hips? You're the pin-up girl for the South Pacific Mangaia Island.

Neck more than a foot long? Great beauty demands it! proclaim the Kayan of Burma.

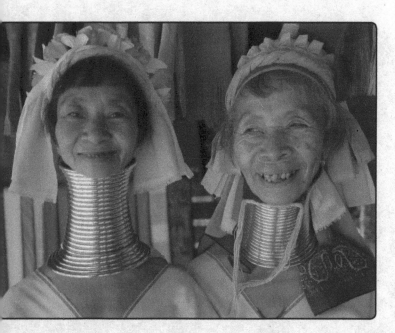

KAYAN WOMEN

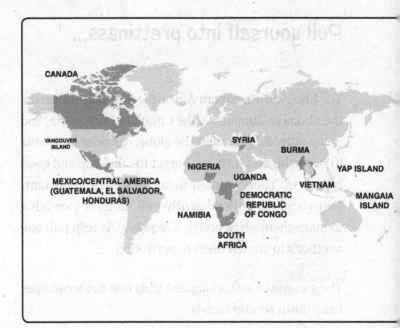

COUNTRIES' IDEAS OF BEAUTY
BURMA; VANCOUVER ISLAND, CANADA; DEMOCRATIC
REPUBLIC OF CONGO; SOUTH AFRICA; MANGAIA;
NAMIBIA; MEXICO/CENTRAL AMERICA (GUATEMALA, EL
SALVADOR, HONDURAS); NIGERIA; SYRIA; UGANDA;
VIETNAM, YAP ISLAND

Pull yourself into prettiness...

The Khoikhoi of southern Africa, the Buganda of Uganda, the Shona in Zimbabwe, the Chuuk in Micronesia, and many other folks around the globe, consider long labia to be the biggest turn-on. Forget the makeup and good hair days. These women focus on what's important. Conscientious girls diligently pull on their own labia to make themselves pretty. Teenage girls help pull one another's to stretch them to perfection.

The gorgeous result: elongated labia that can sometimes hang down several inches.

Some worry all that stretching could be harmful. Young women might pull on the wrong part. And if they don't achieve nice, long labia, their self-image might suffer.

Others say not to worry. It's way safer to lengthen your labia for beauty than to surgically enlarge your breasts (as many Western women do). Plus, there's a major upside: long labia give women more pleasure during sex. All that fun keeps couples loving, marriages intact, and families happy.

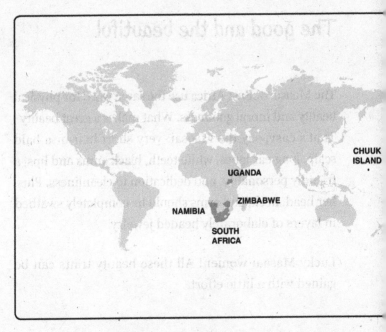

BEAUTY IS LONG LABIA
UGANDA, NAMIBIA, ZIMBABWE, SOUTH AFRICA, CHUUK

The good and the beautiful

The Maasai of East Africa use the same word for physical beauty and moral goodness. What makes a great beauty? That's easy, say the Maasai: very short hair or a bald scalp, long ear lobes, white teeth, black gums and lips, a friendly personality, and dedication to cleanliness. Plus, her head, neck, and arms should be completely swathed in layers of elaborately beaded jewelry.

Lucky Masaai women! All these beauty traits can be gained with a little effort.

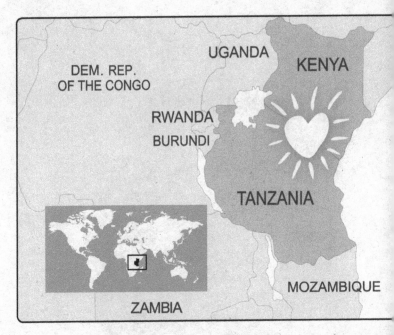

MAASAI OF KENYA AND TANZANIA

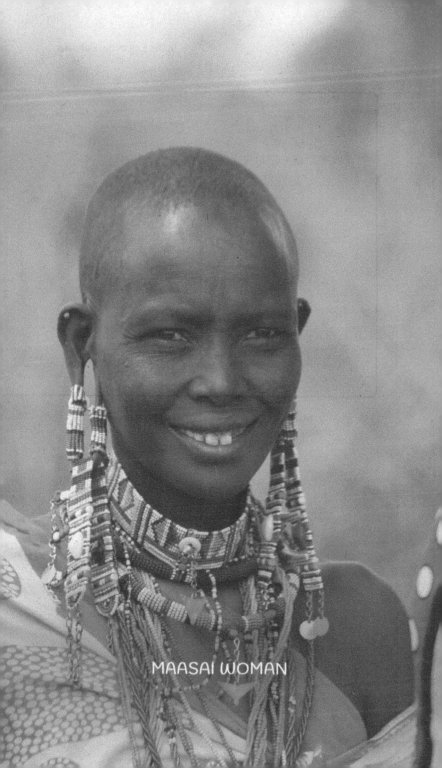

MAASAI WOMAN

IS IT PORN OR IS IT ART?

How important is porn to human beings? This may give you a hint: they began creating it as soon as they figured out tools, more than 10,000 years ago. Archaeologists have found erotic cave paintings dating back to the Paleolithic era.

In ancient India, religious scriptures and sculpture displayed explicitly sexual material. Some of the most beautiful and religious poetry, songs, and visual arts depict highly erotic images. One of the world's most famous "how-tos on sex" is the 2,000-year-old *Kama Sutra*.

In Egypt, archaeologists have found erotica dating back more than 3,000 years.

China maintains its rep as one of the earliest sophisticated cultures. Its extensive erotica dates back more than 1,000 years. Literary and visual erotica thrived and hit a peak in China in the 1600s.

Japan can boast the "world's first novel," The *Tale of Genji*, written by a woman in the eleventh century. It's a *Sex and the City* tale of the hero's many affairs, described in sensual, lustful language. Erotic art continued to flourish in Japan, especially beginning in the 1600s. Some of Japan's most famous artists of the 1800s created beautiful erotic art called *shunga* ("spring pictures").

Westerners were no slouches, either. Erotic sculpture and ceramics were popular in ancient Greece more than 3,000 years ago. Literary porn turned up in Greece dating back to the third century.

The ancient Romans also loved the stuff. Archaeologists have found erotic Roman art dating back more than 2,000 years. Loads of statues, paintings, and even household items were lavishly decorated with sexual themes.

The uptight UK and US lagged behind. They didn't even have a word for porn until the 1800s. The Victorians were scandalized when archaeologists uncovered ancient Roman erotic art in the mid-1800s. They immediately locked the stuff away so as not to corrupt women and the working class. They only allowed scholars – a notoriously undersexed bunch – to see it.

In the nineteenth century, prudes in England, Ireland, and the US got porn outlawed, though they could never clearly explain what it was.

Undeterred, filmmakers began making porn films almost immediately after the invention of motion pictures in the 1890s.

In 1969, Denmark, always a champion of liberty, was the first country to end censorship and thus legalized porn (that showed adults). Despite the First Amendment protecting free speech – and repeated court battles – the US continues to ban porn involving only adults.

The porn controversy will doubtless continue because no one has ever figured out exactly how to define it.

Somewhere on this planet, you're the perfect hunk...

Tired of Saturday nights dateless, horny, and alone? Not to worry. The woman of your dreams is waiting—you just have to look in the right place.

Belly sagging over your belt? Try Great Britain, where many English women prefer men with a paunch.

Fat more in the multi-layers? Head for Nauru, where lots of women go for an obese guy.

Relying on your manly attributes? Sirionó women of eastern Bolivia swoon over long penises.

In some parts of India, short, fat penises are hot.

Not so endowed? In many parts of the world, women agree with the ancient Greeks that large penises are rather gross, and small, firm penises are most appealing.

Tired of being loved only for your pecker? The Maasai women of east Africa are for you. Handsome men, they say, are friendly, self-disciplined, and brave, have good teeth and carry a club. It's also important to be well-dressed, so be sure to wear a bright red cloth wrapped around your hips.

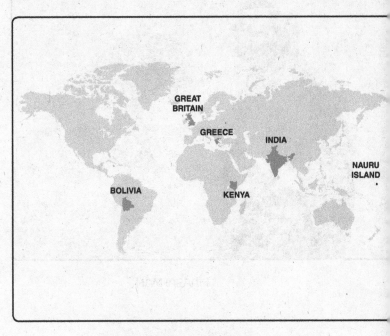

MALE HANDSOMENESS IDEALS
GREAT BRITAIN, GREECE, KENYA, INDIA,
NAURU ISLAND, BOLIVIA

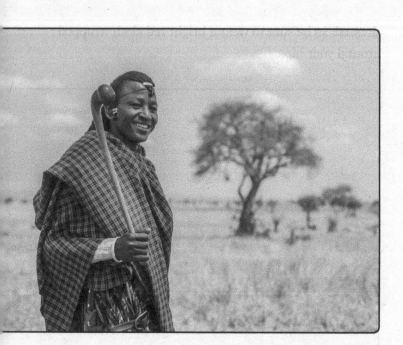

MAASAI MAN

Better start workin' on that tan...

The Akimel O'odham (aka Pima) of the North American Southwest—famous for their artistry, peaceful culture, and ferocious warriors—considered fair skin to be quite ugly. White skin is simply a mistake of the Creator.

The Wogeo of Papua New Guinea regard the light complexion of Europeans—especially blondes—so repulsive it's practically shameful. They understand why Europeans insist on wearing all those clothes—to hide their disgusting pale skin.

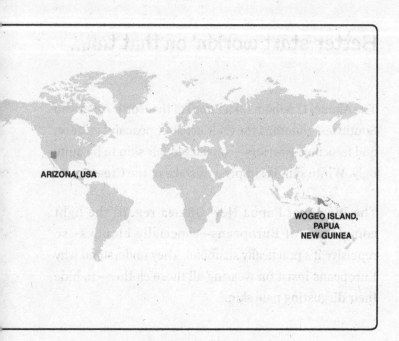

PIMA OF ARIZONA, USA AND
WOGEO OF PAPUA NEW GUINEA

Dieting? Who needs it?

Overweight?

"Impossible!" say lots of folks around the world. Want to look great? Gain a few pounds. Clothes look best when they're taut.

In Fiji, Tonga, Jamaica, and many other countries, jiggly rolls of flab inflame men's desire. Add a few stretch marks and you'll really drive them wild.

In the West African deserts of Niger, the green foothills of southwest Uganda, and hot, humid southeastern Nigeria, women check into a "fattening hut" before marriage. There, they stuff themselves with food to create the bulging silhouette that will make the groom drool. They grow as rotund as possible, to look their very best for the wedding day.

Want to flaunt your corpulence? Join the annual Hangandi Festival Beauty Contest held in the barren, searing deserts of southwest Niger, where women have more babies than anywhere else in the world. But beware—you're competing with seasoned Djerma women who have been chowing down as much sweet and oily food as they can hold, preparing for the event. Only the most enormous, bulging layers of fat will snag the Miss Hangandi crown.

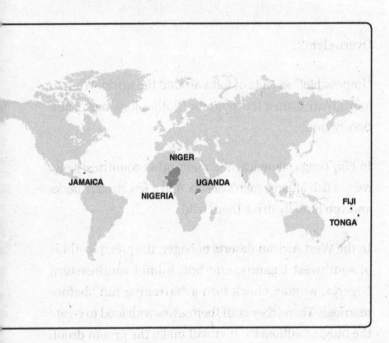

HEAVYWEIGHT BEAUTY
FIJI, TONGA, JAMAICA, NIGER, UGANDA, NIGERIA

Family
TIES

Family. It conjures up myriad images. The "typical" family—Mom, Dad and the kids—is becoming an exotic species, now less than half of US families. Some people still squabble about same-sex marriages and whether kids can be happy with two moms or dads. But how about none? Or one hundred?

What is a "family" anyway? Most of the world considers your "family" to include great-grand-parents, grand-parents, parents, aunts, uncles, sisters, brothers, all cousins, close friends, and their children—and each is responsible for them all.

Where governments are broke and broken, these family ties keep people from growing too poor...or too rich, at least in villages where everyone still knows one another. Few people will wallow in flamboyant luxury while their nephews and nieces are starving or too poor to go to primary school. While you might miss an extra hot car, you gain a wide network of warm relationships.

Misunderstanding people's concept of "family" has derailed many expensive development programs. Take a multi-million dollar family planning program in the Philippines. It created billboards showing two families. On one side stand two parents and two children, dressed in expensive clothes, in front of a large house, with lots of toys in the yard and a new car in the driveway. On the other side are two parents and eight kids. They wear old, worn clothing, some hanging loosely on the smaller children. The parents stand before a bamboo hut with a palm frond roof and glassless windows. No toys, no car. The caption blares confidently, "Which family is happier?"

Months later, the program survey asked that question. The results stunned them. The majority of people replied, "Of course, the happier family is the one with more children." People had seen past the big house, nice clothes, and new car. They knew what made people happy—a large and loving family. They assumed the eight children on the billboard had devoted aunts and uncles, grandparents and friends to help out—even "adopt"—the kids, as needed.

Maybe it is this deep, caring human connection that made the Philippines one of the rare countries to pull off a major, bloodless revolution. In February 1986, hundreds of thousands of people took to the streets, protesting the Marcos dictatorship. For hours, thousands of troops faced the throng. Finally, Marcos commanded the soldiers to fire. They refused. They would not fire on the mothers and fathers, sons and daughters of their neighbors. The Marcos regime fell without a drop of bloodshed, and a new democracy was born.

We can all learn much from the Philippine people.

Four letter words even Grandma wouldn't mind...

Among some aboriginal societies in Australia, the word for man is "penis," woman is "vagina," and children are "semen." So relax when your neighbor calls out cheerily, "Here comes a penis, a vagina, and some semen." She just means a family is strolling down the road.

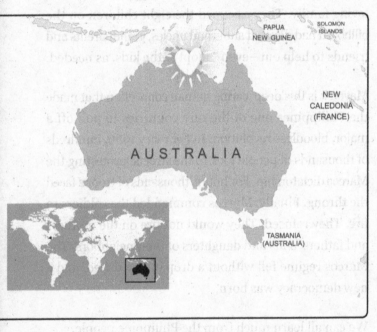

ABORIGINES OF AUSTRALIA

The family that eats together...

Along the fertile banks of the Yuat River and in the dense forests of Papua New Guinea, the Biwat dine on their rich garden produce, plentiful fish, wild game, and...until the 1930s, their neighbors. Of course, they wouldn't eat just anyone. People who spoke the Biwat language were off limits—after all, they could be kin.

But after a successful raid, some creative River Biwat tried chowing down the Bush Biwat people they had captured. To their delight, they found them just as tasty and digestible as anyone else, and so continued to snack on them. That put a definite damper on marriage between the two groups. No one wanted to come home to dinner and find sis and bro were the main course.

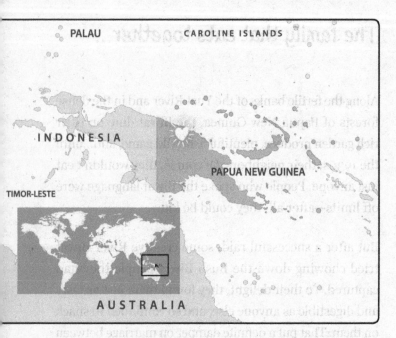

BIWAT OF PAPUA NEW GUINEA

Kissing cousins

The Waorani of Ecuador love their families. There's no one they'd rather live with, hang out with, and party with. Families of eighteen in a house never bicker and certainly never fight. After all, everyone has a right to think what he wants and do as she likes. Why should anyone—man or woman, husband or wife, mom or dad—call the shots for anyone else? *That* would be ridiculous.

What's important is to enjoy life. Hunt with spears and blowguns for food. Laugh, sing, and tell jokes. Keep a good sense of humor. Share what you have. Be kind to your family. And party!

Best are the family parties. Relatives from miles around come to eat, drink, dance, and enjoy new sex-mates among the cousins. Single or married—doesn't matter. Everyone should join the fun.

When it's time to pick a spouse, you have your choice—as long as you choose a cousin or two.

Want to visit? Better hurry. Illegal logging and oil companies are busy destroying the Waorani's forest home.

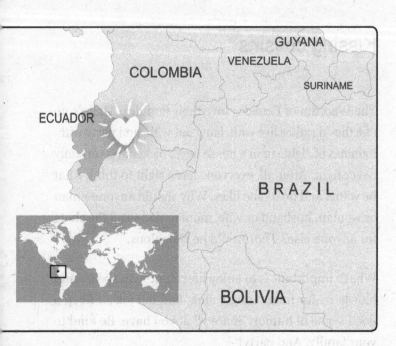

WAORANI OF ECUADOR

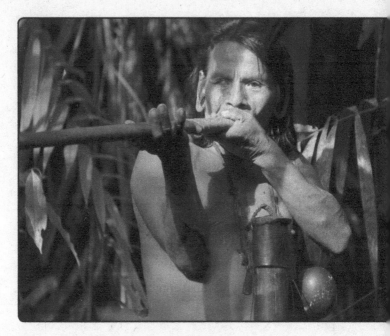

WAORANI MAN WITH BLOWGUN

Hate those dishpan hands?

Constant housework, no right to own land, mother-in-law bosses you around all day. That's life for Khasi men of the northeastern Indian state of Meghalaya ("Home of Clouds").

Khasi families revolve around women. They have all the economic power, are very competitive, and ready to take financial risks. Women pass all land down to their daughters. Her children take her name and, when she marries, her husband must come to live in her mother's home.

Dads are important, too, of course. They keep the house clean, work in the rice fields, sing and play music. They can even work in their wife's or sister's shop, if she permits. Oh, and they can become politicians—as long as they don't interfere with those holding the economic and social power. Sound familiar? Only here, all the top guns are women.

Young men and women have lots of freedom to date, sleep together before marriage, and choose their own spouses. Of course, the man must get approval from his mom and sisters...and from her mom and grandma.

Get pregnant without being married? No problem. The baby takes mom's name anyway and lives like everyone else in mom's home. When a girl is born, everyone cheers and celebrates. Baby is a boy? People politely try to comfort you.

Marry the wrong person? Not to worry. Divorce is easy. Hubby hands his wife five cents, and she gives him a dime, which he throws away. Way easier and cheaper than a divorce lawyer.

These days, some Khasi men are pushing for equal rights. They have even formed an equal rights organization. But most members are anonymous. They don't want their wives or moms to get mad at them.

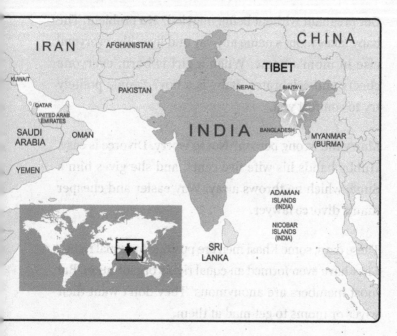

KHASI OF MEGHALAYA, INDIA

WOMEN WHO RULE THE WORLD

Where in the world do women hold the reins of power? In the world's matriarchies, that's where. Check out just a few examples.

Mosuo

One lively group is the Mosuo of China. Mosuo women control the finances, the economic system, businesses, and financial decisions. All property is passed down from moms to daughters. Children grow up in their mom's homes and take her name.

The Mosuo don't bother with formal marriage. Instead they have "walking marriages," where a woman chooses her mate and how long she'll have a relationship with him. During the walking marriage, the women continue to live in their mothers' homes, and the men in *their* mothers' homes.

Think it might be hard to tell who's your papa? You're right. Neither child nor mom may know who the father is – nor does anyone care. What's important is only who mom is. If men want to be involved with children's upbringing, he does it with his sisters' kids.

Minangkabau

The Minangkabau of Indonesia say that mothers are the most important people in the world. In this strongly Islamic society, Minangkabau women rule the households and hold clan property, which they pass down to their daughters. Women also handle the family finances and often own businesses.

According to Minangkabau women and men, they hold equal power, with a division of responsibilities. Men generally handle most of the political and spiritual leadership. Women own all property and many businesses. Although the formal clan chief is always a man, women select the chief and can remove him from office anytime they think he's not doing his job properly. Some women also delve into politics. But women's primary focus is usually to hold and build the family wealth and take care of the future generation of matriarchs.

Akan

The Akan (aka "The Enlightened" or "The Civilized") live in Ghana. In Akan mythology, the origin of the group was a single woman – sort of an Eve without a troublesome Adam.

Akan women have strong economic and political power. All Akan people take their identity, property, wealth, and politics from their mothers. After marriage, a woman remains independent, continues to live in her mom's family, and keeps her economic independence. Women are generally in charge of the all-important industries related to food production, agriculture, fishing, and commerce.

Moms also determine the political lineup. The community elects a top chief ("Ohene") and the queen mother ("Ohemmaa"), who are co-rulers. The *Ohemmaa* is powerful and at times can become "king." She also has primary responsibility for choosing the chief when that spot becomes vacant. Men generally hold major political positions, but they inherit their roles through their mothers and sisters.

Bribri

The Bribri of Costa Rica live in clans led by women. Everyone turns to the wisdom of the natural leaders, the grandmas, who make key decisions based on their knowledge and understanding of tradition.

Thus, women also judge what's ethical and proper, and are the community's spiritual leaders. They are also the only ones able to prep the ingredients that are essential for sacred Bribri rituals. Men can take important roles, too, but they must pass down their knowledge, contacts, and jobs to their sisters' sons, not their own.

Women also have great economic power. Only women can own and inherit land. Girls learn early that they should grow up to be successful businesswomen whose companies support their society and the environment, as well as make money.

Nagovisi

The Nagovisi of South Bougainville Island are led by women. Women own all the land and proudly ensure their land is productive. Although they do get involved in leadership roles and social ceremonies, they keep their eyes on the money, i.e., family land. Women control the food production, and that keeps them independent, and the men reliant on them for food.

Nagovisi don't bother with formal marriages. If she likes a guy, she lets him help her in the garden, sleep with her in her home, and eat her food. It's as close as he'll get to tying the knot with her. If she stops giving him food, he knows they're divorced.

Jarai

The Jarai live in Vietnam, Cambodia, and Laos. Their homes are longhouses, where several close-knit families live together, all linked by the mother. Women inherit property and hand it down to their daughters. Unmarried daughters – and sons – are free to engage in sexual activities, and everyone's fair game except family members.

When a woman is ready to marry, she picks the man she wants. She does the proposing – not on bended knee, but using a matchmaker. The matchmaker informs the lucky guy by giving him a copper bracelet. If he agrees, they get hitched and move into her mom's house. She will own all their property. Their kids become part of her family and will take their mother's family name.

Barbie for boys

Tired of games that teach your sons to maim and kill? Take them to Manus Island, just off Papua New Guinea's north coast. The courageous and skillful Manusians are lords of the Bismark Sea—controlling trade and fishing along the island's south coast.

Manus boys like to learn tough skills as sailors and traders. They also love to play with baby dolls, as anthropologist Margaret Mead discovered. The Manus boys were thrilled when Mead gave each of them a doll. Each boy adored his own dolly and showered it with gentle care. He carried his "baby" everywhere, crooned sweet lullabies, and rocked his dolly tenderly to sleep.

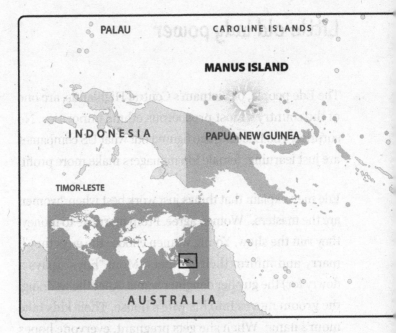

MANUSIANS OF MANUS ISLAND, PAPUA NEW GUINEA

Little old lady power

The Ede people, of Vietnam's Central Highlands, are one of the country's most prosperous ethnic minorities. No surprise. The Ede long ago figured out what US companies are just learning: female top managers make more profit.

Ede men explain that things just work best when "women are the masters." Women agree. From marriage to money, they run the show. Young women choose the guys they'll marry and inform their mothers. Mom "buys" (pays a dowry for) the guy her daughter wants. After the wedding, the groom moves into his wife's house. Their kids take mom's name. When she gets pregnant, everyone hopes for daughters. A son will always be an "outsider," even in his own mom's family.

Women own all of the property, and traditionally are village chiefs, responsible for community affairs, finances, land, and resolving disputes. The oldest Ede woman (*Khoa sang*) is the highest authority in the family and community. Families of four or five generations live together in longhouses, which stand on stilts and have an inside and an outside. The family head woman, her husband, and her married and unmarried daughters get to live inside. Sons have to bed down in the outside room. Women and men must use different staircases—the women's beautifully carved with breasts, the men's plain wood.

But hey, guys aren't just for making babies. Head mom gives them jobs, like dealing with the government and arranging weddings. Whatever he does, though, he must always represent his wife and her family.

If his wife dies, the widower doesn't need to worry that he'll be lonely. His wife's mom and sisters will decide who will marry him next.

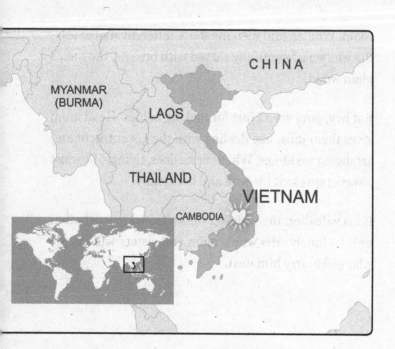

EDE OF VIETNAM

PROTECTING THOSE DELICATE EARS

A recent poll showed that the average person curses about eighty times per day. Shrinks say it's not just common, it's good for you! Studies show that swearing helps reduce pain. One survey found that people who curse a lot are considered more loyal, trustworthy, and upfront with their friends. So swearing is almost as good as eating greens.

Yet some places are determined to protect women's and children's tender psyches by nixing this healthy outlet.

Oklahoma outlaws using "indecent language" in front of either a woman or a child under ten (apparently they are equally vulnerable). Do it, and you could be off to jail for thirty days and pay a $100 fine.

Until 2016, Michigan made it illegal to swear in front of women or children.

In Willowdale, Oregon, it's illegal for a husband to curse while having sex with his wife. Hot damn!

It's wonderful, it's paradise...

In the dense rainforests, thick bamboo groves, and rich agricultural croplands of northern Sumatra, the Atjeh region established the first Muslim royal throne in Indonesia. In the 1600s, Atjeh had four queens (Sultanas Tajul Islam, Nurul Alam, Inayat Shah and Kamalat Shah). For decades, these queens led their courageous troops to defend their homeland against those who tried to impose foreign versions of Islam.

Ordinary Atjehnese women have also been strong. Throughout history, they have tilled farmlands, run households, and raised children, while the men travel far and wide to obtain the things women cannot grow or make.

These Atjehnese women know what paradise is like. It's a wondrous place, with gorgeous trees and perfumed flowers, perfect weather, all kinds of luscious food, and delicious drinks...and no men in sight. The men are traveling out there somewhere, while women enjoy heaven with their women friends, their children, their sisters, and their mothers.

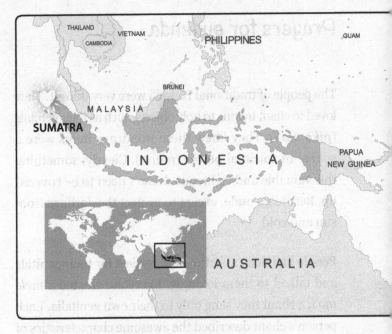

ATJEHNESE OF SUMATRA, INDONESIA

Prayers for pudenda

The people of traditional Hawai'i were very devout. They loved to chant hymns to holy objects, such as their genitals (*piko ma'i*). They knew these wondrous items were a source of spiritual power (*mana*). Clearly, something this valuable and righteous doesn't need to be covered up. Best to go nude, except to protect the darlings from sun and cold.

People had deep affection and respect for their genitals and talked to them lovingly. Everyone created a *mele ma'i*, a chant they sang only to their own genitalia. Each person's chant described the awesome characteristics of his or her sex organs. No room for false humility in these chants. For example, Queen Lili'uokalani (1838-1917) sang of her delightful vulva named "*Anapau*" (Frisky), and how it pranced and danced when it was excited. King Kalākaua (1836-1891) serenaded his penis, lavishing praise on its great size.

These sacred traditions are not entirely lost. Even today, people visit holy Hawaiian sites. There's the huge penis stone and the vulva stone on Moloka'i, and the Vagina Rock, twenty feet long, on the Big Island—great places

for passionate folks to give offerings to improve their
fertility and sexual skills.

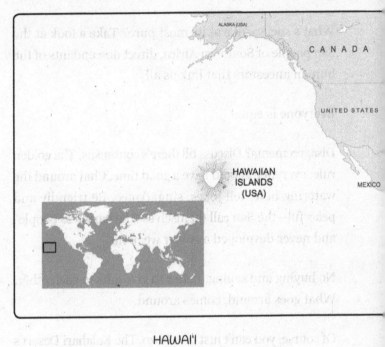

A special kiss on the cheek

What's society like at its most pure? Take a look at the San people of Southern Africa, direct descendants of the human ancestors that link us all.

Everyone is equal.

Disagreements? Discuss till there's consensus. The golden rule: everyone should have a good time. Chat around the watering hole, tell jokes, sing, dance. Be friendly and peaceful—the San call themselves "the harmless people" and never developed any war weapons.

No buying and selling. Better to give gifts to each other. What goes around, comes around.

Of course, you can't just be a Bozo. The Kalahari Desert's a tough hood. Everyone has to bring home the eland meat, wild fruit, and veggies. The San are the ultimate conservationists, know thousands of plants, can track and hunt anywhere.

Ladies, want a nice San dude? Your parents will arrange your first marriage. Don't like their pick? Throw a tantrum. Divorce is easy. Then you can marry anyone and as many times as you like. Another plus: here, getting older really is getting better. Each year, proudly wear your apron a little lower to show your age. The lower the apron, the more respect and authority you have.

Guys, want to marry a charming San lass? If she's never been married, propose to her parents. If they agree and she doesn't, forget it. If she's already divorced and available, give her a kiss on the cheek. Not with your lips, dummy, shoot her in the butt with a small arrow. Just be sure it's not sharp—it should bounce off like a gentle kiss. If she likes you, she'll take it, and you, home. No wedding ceremony needed. But you *will* spend the next eight years working for your in-laws.

Anything annoys you, remember, women control sex. And, as San women observe, men need sex to live.

Plenty to learn from these peaceful, creative folks. But move fast. The San have survived nature's extremes for 22,000 years. But surviving land-grabbing cattle owners and diamond mines is another story.

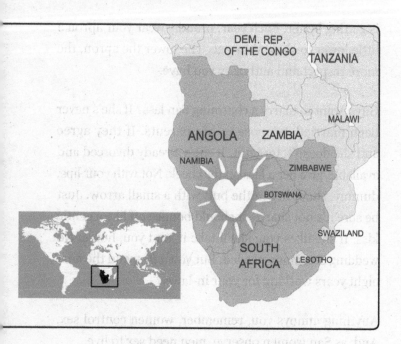

THE SAN OF ANGOLA, BOTSWANA,
NAMIBIA, SOUTH AFRICA, ZIMBABWE

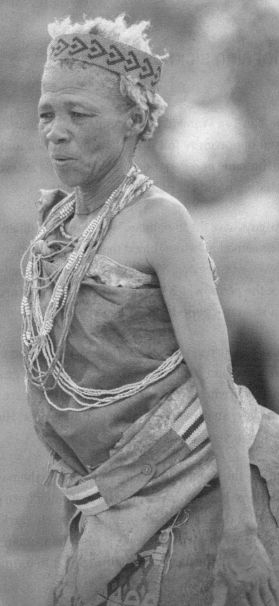

SAN WOMAN

Morning sickness for men

The Tau Taa Wana of Central Sulawesi, Indonesia, are equal opportunity folks. They figure women and men are the same and everyone should get to do everything, including having periods and giving birth.

Yep, guys have the "monthlies," with just a few differences. Their semen is "white" blood that they say is equivalent to women's periods. They also go through rituals that slice the penis, which bleeds to make them mature, just as a woman's periods do for her.

Guys can also get pregnant. Indeed, once upon a time *only* guys had babies. But they moaned and groaned constantly while pregnant. To top it off, they gave birth to measly, unattractive newborns, tiny as ants. Hard to get dewy-eyed over a baby ant.

One day the women got fed up with hearing them whine and offered to take over. Since then, women have given birth. But the guys still get pregnant first. He carries the baby for a week, then inserts it into the woman, who then does all the hard work of bringing it to term. Why are you not surprised?

Don't think the Tau Taa Wana are the only folks who try to get men into the pregnancy act. The Tiwi of the Melville and Bathurst Islands also insist only men can start babies. Guys do it by dreaming of spirit children. Dad tells the dream babe who its mother is, and the baby obediently enters the wife to grow into a human.

There's a payoff of this theory for women. They are relatively free to have extramarital affairs. After all, a woman can only get pregnant through the dreams of her husband, so there's never a question of who's the dad.

Don't feel too smug if you're European. Your recent ancestors had the same idea. The ancient Greeks started it, insisting that only men create babies. Men's semen contain tiny, fully formed humans, which they insert into a woman to grow. Europeans held onto this theory until the seventeenth century, after they figured out how planets move around the sun, how blood circulates through the body, and how to build telescopes.

Some guys will do anything to horn in on the cool things women do.

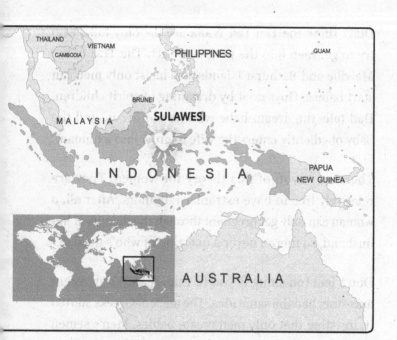

TAU TAA WANA OF SULAWESI, INDONESIA

Sisterly love

The Biwat (aka Mundugumor) live on broad, fertile lands along the Sepik River in Papua New Guinea, rich in coconut trees and sago palms, tobacco fields, lush gardens, and streams teeming with fish. With the livin' so easy, the Biwat have been free to pursue their hobbies—chiefly to make war on their neighbors.

When a Biwat child is born, the parents debate its future. Are they pondering school options and what career to encourage? Nah. They're deciding whether to throw it into the river.

But only the boys are at risk. Girls are much too valuable. Because the only way a Biwat man can get a wife is by trading a sister for her.

Ah, the lucky family with lots of girls! All the sons will have a sister to trade for a wife...unless of course the oldest brother is a greedy SOB and trades all of his sisters for wives for himself. Poor younger brothers—they may end up without a legal wife.

For the man without any sisters to trade, things are grim. Just one way out: try to steal a woman. If the theft succeeds, he must fight her family to keep her. Win that battle, and he gets a shot at enticing her to marry him.

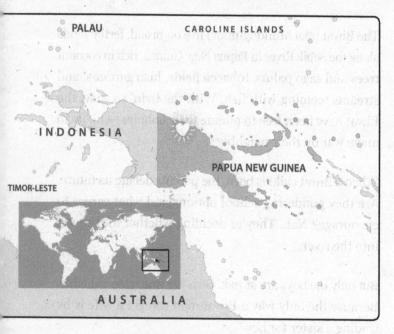

BIWAT OF PAPUA NEW GUINEA

Mother knows best...

The Mosuo (aka the Na) are skilled farmers, growing almost everything they need on their lands among the peaks of the Himalayas in China. The farm animals—water buffalo, horses, geese, chickens—live on the first floor of each family home. Don't be surprised to see a hen march across your bedroom. The second floor is reserved for the women's bedrooms. Everyone else gets to sleep in the attached family "dorm."

Mosuo men gladly live with their mothers and obey her absolutely, throughout their lives—even after they marry. Moms control everything: houses, land, money, livestock, children. But they're benevolent rulers. They take care of the men and encourage them to have hobbies, like playing cards, taking care of the kids, and being town mayor.

Sometimes the men can even help out with real work, when muscle power is needed. Then they happily hand over every cent they make to their moms.

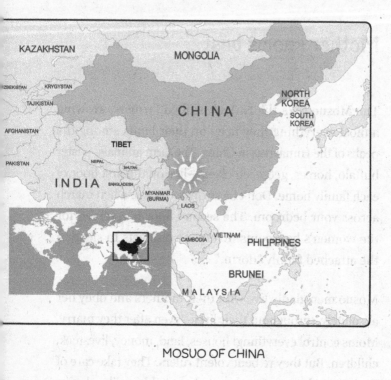

MOSUO OF CHINA

SELECTED Sources

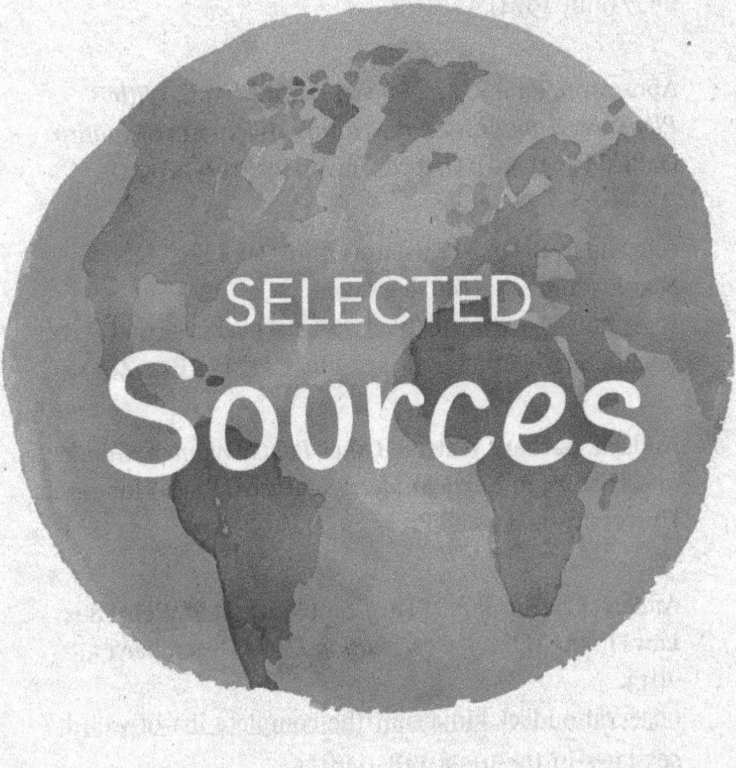

CHAPTER 1. SEX, LIES, AND VIRGINS' TASTES

Abernethy, Virginia. "Dominance and Sexual Behavior: A Hypothesis." *The American Journal of Psychiatry,* 131, no. 7 (July 1974).

Abramson, Paul R. and Steven D. Pinkerton. *With Pleasure: Thoughts on the Nature of Human Sexuality.* Oxford (England): Oxford University Press, 2002.

Alexander, Brian. "Legislating Your Sex Life." *Sexploration* on: NBCNews.com www.nbcnews.com/id/6620768/ns/health-sexual_health/t/legislating-your-sex-life/#.WM3stP21vZ8

Andaya, Barbara Watson. *Other Pasts: Women, Gender and History in Early Modern Southeast Asia.* Honolulu: University of Hawai'i Press, 2001.

Anders, Charlie Jane. "The Complete List of Weird Sex Laws in the U.S.A." *Observation Deck,* December 17, 2013. observationdeck.kinja.com/the-complete-list-of-weird-sex-laws-in-the-u-s-a-1485048155

Beckwith, Carol. "Niger's Wodaabe: People of the Taboo." *National Geographic,* 164, no. 4 (October 1983).

Bovin, Mette. *Nomads who Cultivate Beauty: Wodaabe Dances and Visual Arts in Niger*. Uppsala, Sweden: Nordic Africa Institute, January 2001.

Bullough, Vern L. and Bonnie Bullough, eds. *Human Sexuality: An Encyclopedia*. London and New York: Routledge, 1994.

Buss, David M. *The Evolution Of Desire: Strategies of Human Mating*. New York: Basic Books, 2008.

"Cambodian Love Huts." *National Geographic*. channel.nationalgeographic.com/taboo/videos/cambodian-love-huts/

"Countries and Their Culture: Guajiras." *Every Culture*. www.everyculture.com/wc/Tajikistan-to-imbabwe/Guajiras.html

Corn, David. "The Time Ted Cruz Defended a Ban on Dildos." *Mother Jones*, April 13, 2016. www.motherjones.com/politics/2016/04/ted-cruz-dildo-ban-sex-devices-texas

Côté, James E. "The Implausibility of Freeman's Hoaxing Theory: An Update." *Journal of Youth and Adolescence*, 29, no. 5 (October 2000).

Crocker, William H. "Canela Marriage: Factors in Change." In *Marriage Practices in Lowland South America*, edited by Kenneth M. Kensinger. Urbana and Chicago: University of Illinois Press, 1984.

Crompton, Louis. "An Army of Lovers - The Sacred Band of Thebes." *History Today*, 44, no.11 (November 1994).

Davies, Shary Graham. *Challenging Gender Norms: Five Genders Among Bugis in Indonesia*. Boston: Wadsworth Cengage Learning, September 2006.

Diamond, Milton. "Sexual Behavior in Pre Contact Hawai'i: A Sexological Ethnography." *Revista Española del Pacifico, Pacific Center for Sex and Society,* 2004. www.hawaii.edu/PCSS/biblio/articles/2000to2004 /2004-sexual-behavior-in-pre-contact-hawaii.html

Durex. "Give and Receive: 2005 Global Sex Survey Results." Accessed October 20, 2009. www.data360.org/pdf/20070416064139.Global%20 Sex%20Survey.pdf

Eaves, Ali. "10 Strange Sex Laws That Still Exist!" *Men's Health*. Last modified September 17, 2014. www.menshealth.com/sex-women/10-strange-sex-laws

Elwin, Verrier. *The Muria and Their Ghotul*. Oxford (England): Oxford University Press, 1947.

Ember, Carol R. and Melvin Ember, eds. *Encyclopedia of Sex and Gender - Men and Women in the World's Cultures, Vol. 1 and 2*. New York: Springer Publishing, 2003.

Fallon, Claire. "62 Pet Names Your Honeycake Deserves To Hear On Valentine's Day." *Arts & Culture*. Last modified February 14, 2016. www.huffingtonpost.com/entry/pet-names-foreign-languages_us_56bbbbede4b0c3c5505005ab

Findlaw. statelaws.findlaw.com/

Foreman, Amanda. "The Amazon Women: Is There Any Truth Behind the Myth?" *Smithsonian Magazine*. Last modified April 2014. www.smithsonianmag.com/history/amazon-women-there-any-truth-behind-myth-180950188/

Foster, George M. *Traditional Cultures and the Impact of Technological Change*. New York: Harper & Bros, 1962.

Gagnon, John H. *Human Sexualities*. Scott Foresman and Co., 1977.

"The Gender Issue." *National Geographic*, Jan. 2017.

Giles, G.G., G. Severi, D.R. English, M.R.E. McCredie, R. Borderland, P. Boyle, and J.L. Hopper. "Sexual factors and prostate cancer." *British Journal of Urology International*, 92 (2003): 211-216.

Godelier, Maurice. *The Metamorphoses of Kinship*. New York: Verso Books, 2012.

Golovnev, Andrei V. and Gail Osherenko. *Siberian Survival: The Nenets and Their Story*. Ithaca, NY: Cornell University Press, 1999.

Goodale, Jane Carter and Ann Chowning. *Two-party Line: Conversations in the Field*. Labham, MD: Rowman & Littlefield Publishers, 1996.

Goodenough, Tom. "Cambodian Fathers Build Sex Huts." *Daily Mail*. Last modified July 16, 2012. www.dailymail.co.uk/news/article-2174389/ Cambodian-fathers-build-sex-huts-13-year-old-daughters.html

Graham, Sharyn. "Sex, Gender, and Priests in South Sulawesi, Indonesia." *IIAS Newsletter*, 29, Nov. 2002.

Haake, P., T.H. Krueger, M.U. Goebel, K.M. Heberling, U. Hartmann and M. Schedlowski. "Effects of sexual arousal on lymphocyte subset circulation and cytokine production in man." *Neuroimmunomodulation*, 11 (2004): 293-298.

Harris, Ray. "The Anthropology Of Sex: The Muria Of India." *NovelActivist* (blog), novelactivist.com/926/the-anthropology-of-sex-the-muria-of-india/

Hays, Jeffrey. "Tibetan Marriage, Weddings, Children and Families." *Facts and Details*. Last modified July 2015. factsanddetails.com/china/cat6/sub35/entry-4433.html

Herdt, Gilbert H, ed. *Ritualized Homosexuality in Melanesia (Studies in Melanesian Anthropology)*. Oakland, CA: University of California Press, 1993.

Herdt, Gilbert, ed. *Third Sex, Third Gender: Beyond Sexual Dimorphism in Culture and History*. Cambridge, MA: Zone Books, 1996.

Hurlbert, D. F. and K.E. Whittaker. "The role of masturbation in marital and sexual satisfaction: A comparative study of female masturbators and nonmasturbators." *Journal of Sex Education & Therapy*, 17 (1991): 272-282.

"Iran, Indonesia ban Valentine's Day celebrations." *France24*. Last modified February 14, 2016. www.france24.com/en/20160214-valentine-day-iran-indonesia-ban-celebrations-pakistan-saudi-arabia-february-14

Johnson, Lauren. "Korean Valentine's Year: 12 Romantic Celebrations Every 14th of the Month." *Dumb Little Man Tips for Life*. Last modified January 28, 2017. www.dumblittleman.com/14th-of-every-month-valentine-day/

Kensinger, Kenneth M. *Marriage Practices in Lowland South America (Illinois Studies in Communication)*. Urbana and Chicago: University of Illinois Press, 1984.

Kim, Yvonne. "Valentine's Day in Korea." *Asia Society*. Last modified February 21, 2014. asiasociety.org/korea/valentine%E2%80%99s-day-korea

King, Carol. "40 Spanish Nicknames to Express Affection for Friends, Family, Lovers and Strangers." *Fluent U*. www.fluentu.com/spanish/blog/spanish-nicknames/

King, Chris and Christine Fielder. *Sexual Paradox: Complementarity, Reproductive Conflict and Human Emergence*. Raleigh, NC: Lulu.com, 2006.

Klaw, Spencer. *Without Sin: The Life and Death of the Oneida Community*. New York: Penguin Books, 1994.

Lakshmanan, Indira A.R. "Where Women Rule." *The Boston Globe Magazine*. April 23, 2000.

Lee, Richard B. and Richard Daly, eds. *The Cambridge Encyclopedia of Hunters and Gatherers*. Cambridge (England): Cambridge University Press, 2004.

Lehmiller, Justin. "A Scientist's Response To The 'War On Masturbation.'" *Sex and Psychology*. Last modified March 3, 2014. www.lehmiller.com/blog/2014/3/3/a-scientists-response-to-the-war-on-masturbation

Lepowsky, Maria. *Fruit of the Motherland: Gender in an Egalitarian Society*. New York: Columbia University Press, 1993.

Lewis, Benny. "77 Weird and Romantic Names for the International Lover." *Fluent in 3 Months*. www.fluentin3months.com/valentine/

Lowry, Tara. "The 14th of every month is a holiday in South Korea." *Matador Network*. Last modified February 27, 2013. matadornetwork.com/abroad/the-14th-of-every-month-in-south-korea-is-a-holiday/

Malinowski, Bronislaw. *Sexual Life Of Savages In North-western Melanesia - Ethnographic Account Of Courtship, Marriage & Family Life Among The Natives*. New York: Harvest/Harcourt, Brace & Co, 1929.

Marshall, Donald S. *Human sexual behavior: Variations in the ethnographic spectrum*. New York: Basic Books, 1971.

Marshall, Donald S. "Sexual Behavior in Mangaia." In *Human Sexual Behavior*, edited by Donald S. Marshall and Robert C. Suggs. New York: Basic Books, 1971.

Massachusetts Laws by Subject. www.mass.gov/courts/case-legal-res/law-lib/laws-by-subj/

MacCormack, Carol P. and Marilyn Strathern. *Nature, Culture and Gender*. Cambridge (England): Cambridge University Press, 1980.

McAtear, Olivia. "Here are the 12 most sexually satisfied countries." *Metro*. Last modified May 1, 2015. metro.co.uk/2015/05/01/here-are-the-12-most-sexually-satisfied-countries-5177046/#ixzz4UvkCgO4I

McDowell, Nancy A. "Mundugumor: Sex and Temperament Revisited." In *Being human: An introduction to cultural anthropology*, edited by Mari Womack. Upper Saddle River, NJ: Prentice Hall, 2001.

Mead, Margaret. *Coming of Age in Samoa*. New York: New American Library, 1949.

Mead, Margaret. *Sex and Temperament: In Three Primitive Societies*. New York: W. Morrow & Company, 1935.

Morris, Janet and Chris Morris. *The Sacred Band*. Germantown, TN: Kerlak Enterprises, Inc., 2011.

Morse, Felicity. "Valentine's Day: Countries that don't love February romance." *NewsBeat*. Last modified February 14, 2015. www.bbc.co.uk/newsbeat/article/31382332/valentines-day-countries-that-dont-love-february-romance

"Navajo Cultural Constructs of Gender and Sexuality" posted by kgontarc on *Trans Bodies Across the Globe*, Department of Gender Studies, Indiana University, Bloomington. Last modified December 17, 2010. transgenderglobe.wordpress.com/2010/12/17/navajo-cultural-constructions-of-gender-and-sexuality/

Oestmoen, Per Inge. "Women in Mongol society." *Cold Siberia*. Last modified January 23, 2001. www.coldsiberia.org/monwomen.htm

Oliver, Douglas L. *Oceania: The Native Cultures of Australia and the Pacific Islands*. Honolulu: University of Hawai'i Press, 1989.

Pinkerton, S. D., L.M. Bogart, H. Cecil, and P.R. Abramson. "Factors associated with masturbation in a collegiate sample." *Journal of Psychology & Human Sexuality*, 14 (2003): 103-121.

Porath, Jason. "Khutulun (1260-1306)." *Rejected Princesses*.
www.rejectedprincesses.com/princesses/khutulun

Qin, Amy. "'Kingdom of Daughters' in China Draws Tourists to Its Matrilineal Society." *New York Times* (New York, NY), Oct. 25, 2015.

Passell, Lauren. "82 Ridiculous (Real) Laws That Could Screw Up Your Love Life." *The Date Report*.
www.thedatereport.com/dating/buzzkills/dumb-us-laws-sex-love/

Randell, John. *Sexual Variations*. Boca Raton, Florida: CRC Press, 1976.

Reese, Lyn. "Mongolian Women." *Women in World History*.
www.womeninworldhistory.com/mongolian8.html

Richinick, Michele. "Guns in Georgia town: OK. Sex toys: Not so much." *MSNBC*. Last modified May 22, 2014.
www.msnbc.com/msnbc/georgia-city-sex-toy-law-lawsuits

Rollin, Betty. "Motherhood – Who Needs It?" *Look*, 34, no. 19 (1970).

Rosaldo, Michelle Zimbalist. "A Theoretical Overview." In *Woman, Culture and Society,* edited by Michelle Zimbalist Rosaldo and Louise Lampere. Stanford, CA: Stanford University Press, 1974.

Rotherman, Joshua. "The Real Amazons." *The New Yorker*. Last modified October 17, 2014. www.newyorker.com/books/joshua-rothman/real-amazons

"Satisfaction in Having Sex by Country." *ChartsBin.com*. Accessed January 5, 2017. chartsbin.com/view/4f8

Shankar, Sondeep. "Return of the ritual." *India Today*. Last modified June 30, 1997. indiatoday.intoday.in/story/controversial-custom-of-teenage-mating-among-muria-tribals-gains-ground-in-madhya-pradesh/1/277245.html

Skerritt, Anjella E. *Free to Be Sexually Safe: Empowered to Be Aware and Take Action at All Ages*. Bloomington, Indiana: iUniverse, 2012.

Smith, Jessica. "16 Valentine's Day Traditions From Around The World." *BoredPanda*. www.boredpanda.com/valentines-day-traditions-around-world-vashi/

Styles, Ruth. "Inside the World's Original Free Love Community." *Daily Mail*. Last modified May 14, 2014. www.dailymail.co.uk/femail/article-2627148/Inside-worlds-original-free-love-community-Trobriand-Islanders-change-spouses-want-dedicated-love-huts-settle-differences-game-cricket.html

Taylor, Alan. "The Nenets of Siberia." *The Atlantic*. Last modified April 11, 2012. www.theatlantic.com/photo/2012/04/the-nenets-of-siberia/100277/

"Waorani - Marriage and Family." *Countries and Their Cultures*. www.everyculture.com/South-America/Waorani-Marriage-and-Family.html

Ward, Marguerite. "Sweet Ways People Across the World Celebrate Valentine's Day." *Mic*. Last modified February 14, 2014. mic.com/articles/82361/sweet-ways-people-across-the-world-celebrate-valentine-s-day#.YNtAnZod2

Ward, Martha and Monica Edenstein. *A World Full of Women*. Boston: Pearson, 2009.

Watkins, Joanne C. *Spirited Women*. New York: Columbia University Press, 1996.

Watson, Lawrence C. "Marriage and Sexual Adjustment in Guajira Society." *Ethnology*, 12, no. 2 (1973).

Wayland-Smith, Ellen. *Oneida: From Free Love Utopia to the Well-Set Table*. New York: Picador, 2016.

Wayuu People, *Wikipedia*.
en.wikipedia.org/wiki/Wayuu_people

Wilford, John Noble. "Sexes Equal on South Sea Isle," *New York Times* (New York, NY), March 29, 1994.

Wylie, Kevan. "A Global Survey of Sexual Behaviors." *Porterbrook Clinic*. Last modified April 2009.
www.researchgate.net/publication/228641949_A_Global_Survey_of_Sexual_Behaviours

Wolman, Benjamin B. and John Money. *Handbook of Human Sexuality*. Lanham, MD: Jason Aronson, 1993.

Worrall, Simon. "Amazon Warriors Did Indeed Fight and Die Like Men." *National Geographic*. Last modified October 28, 2014.
news.nationalgeographic.com/news/2014/10/141029-amazons-scythians-hunger-games-herodotus-ice-princess-tattoo-cannabis/

CHAPTER 2. MARRIAGE AND OTHER MYSTERIES

Ager, Lynn Price. "The Economic Role of Women in Alaskan Eskimo Society." In *A World of Women,* edited by Erika Bourguignon. New York: Praeger, 1980.

Bonvillain, Nancy. *Native Nations: Cultures and Histories of Native North America.* Lanham, MD: Rowman & Littlefield, 2016.

Broude, Gwen J. "Extramarital sex norms in cross-cultural perspective." *Behavior Science Research,* 15, no. 3 (1980).

Broude, Gwen J. "Variations in Sexual Attitudes, Norms, and Practices." *In New Directions in Anthropology,* edited by Carol R. Ember, Melvin R. Ember, and Peter N. Peregrine. Boston: Pearson, 2003.

Crooks, Robert L. and Karla Baur. *Our Sexuality.* Boston: Wadsworth Cengage Learning, 2016.

Ember, Carol R. and Melvin Ember, eds. *Encyclopedia of Sex and Gender - Men and Women in the World's Cultures, Vol. 1 and 2.* New York: Springer Publishing, 2003.

FindLaw.
statelaws.findlaw.com

Fisher, Helen E. *Anatomy of Love: A Natural History of Mating, Marriage, and Why We Stray*. New York: W. W. Norton & Company, 2016.

Foster, Peter. "Film star faces lawsuit after 'marrying' a tree." *Telegraph*. Last modified February 1, 2007. www.telegraph.co.uk/news/worldnews/1541309/Film-star-faces-lawsuit-after-marrying-a-tree.html

Gorer, Geoffrey. *Himalayan Village*. Gloucestershire (United Kingdom): Alan Sutton, 1984.

Haworth Abigail. "Why Straight Women Are Marrying Each Other." *Marie Claire*. Last modified July 25, 2016. www.marieclaire.com/culture/a21668/the-tanzanian-wives/

Hennigh, Lawrence. *Functions and Limitations of Alaskan Eskimo Wife Trading*. http://pubs.aina.ucalgary.ca/arctic/arctic23-1-24.pdf.

Hunter, Monica. *Reaction to Conquest Effects of Contact With Europeans on the Pondo of South Africa*. Oxford (England): Oxford University Press, 1961.

Ingoldsby, Bron B. and Suzanna D Smith, eds. *Families in Global and Multicultural Perspective*. Thousand Oaks, CA: SAGE, 2006.

Ipellie, Alootook. "Walking Both Sides of an Invisible Border." *IsumaTV*. www.isuma.tv/journals-knud-rasmussen-sense-memory-and-high-definition-inuit-storytelling/journals-knud-rasmussen

Krige, Jensen E. and J.D. Krige. *The Realm of a Rain Queen: a Study of the Pattern of Lovedu Society*. Oxford (England): Oxford University Press, 1947.

Leacock, Eleanor Burke. *Myths of male dominance: Collected articles on women cross-culturally*. New York: Monthly Review Press, 1981.

Moral, Beatriz. "Erotic Legends and Narratives in Chuuk, Micronesia." *Micronesian Journal of the Humanities and Social Sciences*, 1, no. 1-2 (December 2002).

Morris, John. *Living with Lepchas: A Book About the Sikkim Himalayas*. London: W. Heinemann Ltd, 1938.

Nash, Jill. "Women and Power in Nagovisi Society." *Journal de la Société des océanistes*, 34, no. 60 (1978). www.persee.fr/doc/jso_0300-953x_1978_num_34_60_2974

Nash, Jill. "Women, Work and Change in Nagovisi."
In *Rethinking Women's Roles: Perspectives from the
Pacific,* edited by Denise O'Brien and Sharon W. Tiffany.
Oakland, CA: University of California Press, 1984.

Powdermaker, Hortense. *Life in Lesu: The Study of
Melanesian Society in New Ireland.* New York: W. W.
Norton & Company, 1971.

Rosaldo, Michelle Zimbalist and Louise Lamphere, eds.
Women, Culture and Society. Stanford, CA: Stanford
University Press, 1974.

Rubel, Arthur J. "Partnership and Wife-Exchange
Among the Eskimo and Aleut of Northern North
America." *Anthropological Papers of the University of
Alaska,* 10, No. 1.
www.uaf.edu/files/apua/Rubel1961.pdf

Sachs, Karen. "Engels Revisited: Women, the
Organization of Production, and Private Property."
In *Woman, Culture and Society,* edited by Michelle
Zimbalist Rosaldo and Louise Lampere. Stanford:
Stanford University Press, 1974.

Samimi, Mehrnaz. "Online 'Sigheh'in Iran:
Revolutionary or Restricting?" *Huffington Post.*
www.huffingtonpost.com/mehrnaz-samimi/online-
sighehin-iran-revo_b_6182110.html

Samuels, Gabriel. "Straight Women in Tanzania Marry Each Other in Order to Keep Their Houses." *Independent*. Last modified July 29, 2016. www.independent.co.uk/news/world/africa/straight-women-kurya-tanzania-africa-married-property-domestic-violence-fgm-a7162066.html

Sciolino, Elaine. "Love Finds a Way in Iran: 'Temporary Marriage'." *New York Times* (New York, NY), October 4, 2000.

Sfetcu, Nicolae. *Dating and Interpersonal Relationships*. Nicolae Sfetcu, 2014.

Shams, Daniel. "Matriarchal Societies Nagovisi, Khasi, Garo, Machiguenga." *HELIOTRICITY*. www.heliotricity.com/matriarchalsocieties.html

Singh, Amardeep. "Aishwarya Marries Tree(s)--A Setback for Feminism?" *Amardeep Singh* (blog). Last modified February 6, 2007. www.lehigh.edu/~amsp/2007/02/aishwarya-marries-trees-setback-for.html

Smedley, Audrey. *Women Creating Patrilyny: Gender and Environment in West Africa*. Lanham, MD: Rowman Altamira Press, 2004.

Tanner, Nancy. "Matrifocality in Indonesia and Africa and Among Black Americans." In *Woman, Culture and Society,* edited by Michelle Zimbalist Rosaldo and Louise Lamphere. Stanford: Stanford University Press, 1974.

WomensDay Staff. "10 Obscure Marriage Laws in the U.S." *Woman's Day.* Last modified August 16, 2010. www.womansday.com/relationships/dating-marriage/advice/a1846/10-obscure-marriage-laws-in-the-us-110196/

Wolman, Benjamin B. and John Money. *Handbook of Human Sexuality.* Lanham, MD: Jason Aronson, 1993.

CHAPTER 3. FOXY LAD(Y)

Brame, Gloria G., William D. Brame and Jon Jacobs. *Different Loving: The World of Sexual Dominance and Submission.* New York: Villard, 1996.

Breidlid, Anders, ed. *A Concise History of South Sudan.* Kampala, Uganda: Fountain Publishers, 2014.

Buchli, Victor. *Material Culture: Critical Concepts In The Social Sciences.* London and New York: Routledge, 2004.

"Dinka of Sudan." *FUTURE SEED OF SUDAN*.
futureseed.weebly.com/culture-and-people.html

Fadlalla, Mohamed Hassan. *Customary Laws in
Southern Sudan: Customary Laws of Dinka and Nuer*.
Bloomington, Indiana: iUniverse, 2009.

Francoeur, Robert T. and Raymond J. Noonan, eds. *The
Continuum Complete International Encyclopedia of
Sexuality*. London: A&C Black, 2004.

Levy, Robert I. "The Community Function of Tahitian
Male Transvestitism." *Anthropological Quarterly*, 44,
(January 1971).

Michaels, Axel and Christoph Wulf, eds. *Images of the
Body in India: South Asian and European Perspectives
on Rituals and Performativity*. London and New York:
Routledge India, 2016.

"19th Century Nguni Prepuce Covers." *Gallery
Ezakwantu*.
archive.is/MbKEd#selection-589.0-597.28

Nocentelli, Carmen. *Empires of Love: Europe, Asia, and
the Making of Early Modern Identity*. Philadelphia, PA:
University of Pennsylvania Press, 2013.

"Odd State Laws." *Harford Community College*. https://ww2.harford.edu/faculty/DVolkart/Handouts/ odd_state_laws.htm

"People Profile: The Dinka of South Sudan." *Virtual Research Centre*. www.strategyleader.org/profiles/dinka.html

Rosaldo, Michelle Zimbalist and Louise Lamphere, eds. *Women, Culture and Society*. Stanford, CA: Stanford University Press, 1974.

Russell, Rebecca Ross. *Gender and Jewelry: A Feminist Analysis*. CreateSpace Independent Publishing Platform, 2010.

Saadawi, Nawal El. *The Hidden Face of Eve: Women in the Arab World*. London: Zed Books, 2007.

Stanley, David. *Tahiti-Polynesia Handbook*. Berkeley, CA: Avalon Travel Publishing, 1989.

Ucko, Peter J. *Penis Sheaths: A Comparative Study*. London: Royal Anthropological Institute of Great Britain and Ireland, 1969.

Waldman, Carl and Molly Braun. *Atlas of the North American Indian*. New York: Infobase Publishing, 2009.

CHAPTER 4. IN THE EYE OF THE BEHOLDER

Albers, Susan. "Fat Is Beautiful." *Huffington Post*. Last modified May 25, 2011. www.huffingtonpost.com/dr-susan-albers/fat-is-beautiful_b_526534.html

Ardren, Traci and Scott R. Hutson, eds. *The Social Experience of Childhood in Ancient Mesoamerica*. Boulder, CO: University Press of Colorado, 2006

Berghe, Pierre L. van den and Peter Frost. "Skin Color Preference, Sexual Dimorphism and Sexual Selection." *Ethnic and Racial Studies,* 9, no. 1 (1986).

Cox, Tracey. "Good News, Guys!" *Daily Mail*. Last modified December 3, 2013. www.dailymail.co.uk/femail/article-2741786/Good-news-guys-Over-75-women-prefer-FLAB-abs-Sex-therapist-Tracey-Cox-explains-women-DON-T-want-chiselled-perfection-bed.html

Ember, Carol R. and Melvin Ember, eds. *Encyclopedia of Sex and Gender - Men and Women in the World's Cultures, Vol. 1 and 2*. New York: Springer Publishing, 2003.

Folakemiodoaje. "African Women and Pleasure," *Folakemi*. Last modified September 30, 2014. www.folakemiodoaje.com/2014/09/30/african-women-quest-for-sexual-pleasure/

Goldhill, Simon. *Love, Sex & Tragedy: How the Ancient World Shapes Our Lives*. Chicago, IL: University Of Chicago Press, 2005.

Haleauganda. "Elongation: Okukyalira Ensiko, the Buganda way of enhancing sexual pleasure," Humanist Uganda. Last modified May 21, 2012. humanistuganda.wordpress.com/2012/05/21/elongation-okukyalira-ensiko-the-buganda-way-of-enhancing-sexual-pleasure/

Holmberg, Allan R. *Nomads of the Long Bow*. Washington, DC: Smithsonian Institution, 1950.

Hyde, Montgomery. *A History of Pornography*. New York: Farrar, Straus and Giroux (FSG), 1964.

Koster, Marian and Lisa Leimar Price. "Rwandan Female Genital Modification." In *Culture, Health & Sexuality*, edited by Peter Aggleton, Richard Parker, and Felicity Thomas. London and New York: Routledge, 2015.

Martens, Michael. *Tooth Transfigurement in Indonesia*. Sulawesi Language Alliance, 2013. sulang.org/sites/default/files/sulanglextopics017-v1.pdf

Neff, Mary L. "Pima and Papago Legends." *Journal of American Folklore,* 25 (January 1, 1912).

Saunders, Margaret O. "Women's Role in a Muslim Hausa Town." In *A World of Women,* edited by Erika Bourguignon. New York: Praeger, 1980.

Swami, Viren and Martin J. Tove. "Does Hunger Influence Judgments of Female Physical Attractiveness?" *British Journal of Psychology,* 97 (August 2006).

Promchertchoo, Pichayada. "Ancient Tradition of Long-neck Women Fades as Myanmar Develops." *Channel News Asia.* Last modified December 8, 2016. www.channelnewsasia.com/news/asiapacific/ancient-tradition-of-long-neck-women-fades-as-myanmar-develops/3347404.html

Willcox, Katie H. *Healthy Is the New Skinny: Your Guide to Self-Love in a "Picture Perfect" World.* Carlsbad, CA: Hay House, Inc, 2017.

CHAPTER 5. FAMILY TIES

Atkinson, Jane Monnig and Shelly Errington, eds. *Power and Difference: Gender in Island Southeast Asia.* Stanford, CA: Stanford University Press, 1990.

Berndt, Ronald M. *Love Songs of Arnhem Land*. Chicago: University of Chicago Press, 1978.

Bouissou, Julien. "Where Women of India Rule the Roost and Men Demand Gender Equality." *The Guardian*. Last modified January 18, 2011. www.theguardian.com/world/2011/jan/18/india-khasi-women-politics-bouissou

Burton, Neal. "Hell Yes: The 7 Best Reasons for Swearing." *Psychology Today*. Last modified May 19, 2012. www.psychologytoday.com/blog/hide-and-seek/201205/hell-yes-the-7-best-reasons-swearing

Chodorow, Nancy. "Family Structure and Feminine Personality." In *Woman, Culture and Society*, edited by Michelle Zimbalist Rosaldo and Louise Lamphere. Stanford, CA: Stanford University Press, 1974.

Diamond, Milton. "Sexual Behavior in Pre Contact Hawai'i: A Sexological Ethnography." *Revista Española del Pacífico, Pacific Center for Sex and Society*. Last modified October 4, 2009. www.hawaii.edu/PCSS/biblio/articles/2000to2004/2004-sexual-behavior-in-pre-contact-hawaii.html

Ember, Carol R. and Melvin Ember, eds. *Encyclopedia of Sex and Gender - Men and Women in the World's Cultures, Vol. 1 and 2*. New York: Springer Publishing, 2003.

"Gender Roles of Women of the Ede People in Vietnam." *Cross-cultural Perspectives on Sexuality*. May 3, 2014. www.crossculturalsexuality.wikispaces.com/ Gender+Roles+of+Women+of+the+Ede+People+in +Vietnam

Godelier, Maurice. *The Metamorphoses of Kinship*. New York: Verso Books, 2012.

Lakshmanan, Indira A.R. "Where Women Rule." *The Boston Globe Magazine*. April 23, 2000.

Lamphere, Louise. "Strategies, Cooperation and Conflict Among Women in Domestic Groups." In *Woman, Culture and Society*, edited by Michelle Zimbalist Rosaldo and Louise Lamphere. Stanford, CA: Stanford University Press, 1974.

Leacock, Eleanor. "Women's Status in Egalitarian Society: Implications for Social Evolution." *Current Anthropology*, 19, no. 2 (June 1978).

Lee, Richard B. "What Hunters Do for a Living, Or, How to Make Out on Scarce Resources." In *Man the Hunter*, edited by Richard B. Lee and Irven DeVore. Chicago: Aldine Publishing Company, 1968.

Marsh, Amy. "Le'ale'a O Na Poe Kahiko - Joy of the People of Old Hawai'i." *Electronic Journal of Human Sexuality,* 14 (February 14, 2011). www.ejhs.org/volume14/Joy.htm

"Matriarchies Around the World." *Maps of the World.* www.mapsofworld.com/around-the-world/matriarchy. html

Mead, Margaret. *Sex and Temperament: In Three Primitive Societies.* New York: W. Morrow & Company, 1935.

McDowell, Nancy A. "Mundugumor: Sex and Temperament Revisited." In *Being human: An introduction to cultural anthropology*, edited by Mari Womack. Upper Saddle River, NJ: Prentice Hall, 2001.

Ndoro, Gloria. "Viable matriarchal societies in a modern world prevalent with patriarchy." *Makamba Online.* Last modified April 15, 2016. www.makambaonline.com/index.php/2016/04/15/ viable-matriarchal-societies-in-a-modern-world- prevalent-with-patriarchy/#.WM8RD_21tiM

Qin, Amy. "'Kingdom of Daughters' in China Draws Tourists to Its Matrilineal Society." *New York Times* (New York, NY), October 25, 2015.

Sears, Laurie Jo, ed. *Fantasizing the Feminine in Indonesia*. Durham, NC: Duke University Press Books, 1996.

Sen, Soumen. *Folklore Identity Development In the Context of North-East India*. Kolkata, India: Anjali Publishers, 2013.

Siegel, James T. *The Rope of God*. Ann Arbor, MI: University of Michigan Press, 2000.

Tanner, Nancy. "Matrifocality in Indonesia and Africa and Among Black Americans." In *Woman, Culture and Society*, edited by Michelle Zimbalist Rosaldo and Louise Lamphere. Stanford, CA: Stanford University Press, 1974.

Victor, Daniel. "Women in Company Leadership Tied to Stronger Profits, Study Says." *New York Times* (New York, NY), February 9, 2016.

Walsh, Richard T. and Dr. Barbara Poremba. *Ethnic Minorities of Vietnam*. Salem State University, 1999. w3.salemstate.edu/%7Ebporemba/vietnam/minorities. html

"Waorani - Marriage and Family." *Countries and Their Cultures*.
www.everyculture.com/South-America/Waorani-Marriage-and-Family.html

Ward, Martha, and Monica Edenstein. *A World Full of Women*. Boston: Pearson, 2009.

Wen, Tiffanie. "The Surprising Benefits of Swearing."
BBC. Last modified March 3, 2016.
www.bbc.com/future/story/20160303-the-surprising-benefits-of-swearing

Printed in the USA
CPSIA information can be obtained
at www.ICGtesting.com
JSHW031318210823
46931JS00006B/296

9 781633 535930